"'Just don't do it' isn't enough. Let's face it. Today's young people chronically encounter sexually charged images and messages, but rarely hear the whole story. They are looking for real answers to tough questions, and *Sex Matters* isn't afraid to tell them the unedited truth. Every teenager with an Internet connection or a phone in their pocket needs to read this book!"

—Doug Fields, co-founder of DownloadYouthMinistry.com, youth pastor for thirty years at Saddleback & Mariners Church, speaker, and author of 50+ books including *7 Ways to Be Her Hero*

"As a youth pastor I'm so grateful for Jonathan and his straightforward, honest approach to sexuality and the pressures facing students today. The topics addressed and the real-life case studies hit to the heart of where kids are today. This isn't a sanitized, Christianized, moralized 'just say no' approach but a practical approach to what's really pressuring kids today with biblical wisdom for how to succeed. This is one book that every parent, student, and youth pastor needs on their shelf. *Sex Matters* has been added to my short list of books every parent and student needs to read before leaving middle school . . . yup, middle school."

—Pete Sutton, director of student ministry and middle school pastor, Christ Community Church, St. Charles, Illinois

"This could be the most honest and relevant book available for teenagers in your ministry. I wish I had something this honest and helpful in my hands when I was a teenager."

—Brooklyn Lindsey, youth minister, Nazarene Youth International and ReThink Group; author, *99 Thoughts for Junior High* and *Confessions of a Not-So-Supermodel*

"There are a lot of potentially embarrassing questions that rattle around the minds of many Christian teenagers when it comes to sex (*How far is too far? Is masturbation a sin?* stuff like that). Using powerful stories, eye-opening facts, and surprisingly blunt biblical truth, Jonathan McKee answers these kinds of tough questions with the right mix of truth and grace. He gives teenagers a clear path to living a pure life in a sex-saturated world. Get it, read it, and learn how to let your life and light shine in the darkness."

—Greg Stier, president, Dare 2 Share (www.dare2share.org)

"*Sex Matters* provides super-helpful, truthful answers to the big questions you've wondered about, but never asked. Way better than anything you'll find through a web search."

—Scott Rubin, junior high pastor,
Willow Creek Community Church

"Every great adventure starts with preparation. Sex is a great adventure! But it requires thoughtful preparation. Jonathan McKee's *Sex Matters* is the perfect tool to prepare you for that journey. Do yourself a favor and spend some time thinking, processing, and preparing for the great adventure of sex."

—Josh Griffin, Founder of DownloadYouthMinistry.com
and high school pastor at Saddleback Church

SEX MATTERS

Books by Jonathan McKee
from Bethany House Publishers

Get Your Teenager Talking
More Than Just the Talk
Sex Matters

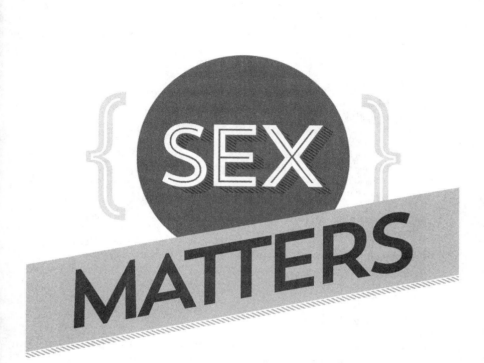

JONATHAN MCKEE

BETHANYHOUSEPUBLISHERS

a division of Baker Publishing Group
Minneapolis, Minnesota

Published by Bethany House Publishers
11400 Hampshire Avenue South
Bloomington, Minnesota 55438
www.bethanyhouse.com

Bethany House Publishers is a division of
Baker Publishing Group, Grand Rapids, Michigan

Printed in the United States of America

Library of Congress Cataloging-in-Publication Data is on file at the Library of Congress, Washington, DC.

ISBN 978-0-7642-2213-9

Unless otherwise indicated, Scripture quotations are from the *Holy Bible*, New Living Translation, copyright © 1996, 2004, 2007 by Tyndale House Foundation. Used by permission of Tyndale House Publishers, Inc., Carol Stream, Illinois 60188. All rights reserved.

Scripture quotations identified NIV are from the Holy Bible, New International Version®. NIV®. Copyright © 1973, 1978, 1984, 2011 by Biblica, Inc.™ Used by permission of Zondervan. All rights reserved worldwide. www.zondervan.com

Scripture quotations identified NIV 1984 are from the HOLY BIBLE, NEW INTERNATIONAL VERSION®. Copyright © 1973, 1978, 1984 Biblica. Used by permission of Zondervan. All rights reserved.

Some names and details have been changed to protect the privacy of those whose stories appear in this book.

Cover design by Greg Jackson, Thinkpen Design, Inc.

Author is represented by WordServe Literary Group.

15   16   17   18   19   20   21   7   6   5   4   3   2   1

Contents

Acknowledgments

don't think I've ever requested as much feedback from friends as I did with this book. This subject always catalyzes a wide array of responses, so I solicited the help of numerous friends, other authors, parents, and youth workers to help me ensure a message relevant to today's young people.

Thanks to Brian Berry, Pete Sutton, and my brother Thom, who all poured over this book in detail, offering helpful feedback and tweaks. Thanks to Julie Smith, Sande Quattlebaum, Jennifer Smith, Rick Nier, and Joe and Kerry Vivian. Your insights as parents were extremely helpful. Thanks to so many of my blog readers at JonathanMcKeeWrites.com who sent in common questions they hear from young people. And thanks to the many friends and colleagues in the field of parenting and youth ministry who read this book and offered the kind endorsements you see in the first few pages.

Thanks to my friend and agent Greg Johnson from Word-Serve for making this project happen. Thanks to Andy, Carra, Ellen, and the entire team at Bethany for your hard work on this book, helping make it a practical tool to put in the hands of young people, parents, and youth workers.

And thanks mostly to my family for supporting me through this project, putting up with my endless questions and prodding about the subject. You guys rock!

But anything truly good that appears on these pages is from God, who deserves all the credit. God, thanks for your amazing design of sex and intimacy! It's mind-boggling why we constantly mess it up. Thanks for enduring with us when we do. We don't deserve your undeniable love and grace.

A Note to Parents Who Might Be Screening This Book

I've never met a parent who engaged in conversations with their kids about sex *too much*.

Not one. Ever.

But in over twenty years of youth ministry, and a decade of writing and speaking to parents, I've met thousands of parents who have done the exact opposite and looked back in regret: *I wish I would have engaged in more of these dialogues.*

Similarly, I've never met a parent who stirred up unhealthy thoughts about sex in their young teen's mind when they engaged in a conversation about what the Bible says about sex. Teenagers don't hear a verse from Proverbs and start thinking lustful thoughts. TV, YouTube, and the phones in their pockets usually provide enough of those distractions.

Some parents think, *My kids aren't thinking about this yet,* so they remain silent. Meanwhile, almost every other voice in their kids' ears feeds them lies about sex. If you want a sample, just Google the lyrics of the songs they hear repeatedly, or sit down and take a peek at any of the images they readily encounter on the screens they stare at for literally hours each day. Or next time you're at the grocery store checkout line, look at the magazine headlines to your right and your left. Do you think your kids haven't noticed those?

As a parent of three kids, ages seventeen, nineteen, and twenty-one, I sincerely wish they didn't have to endure these distractions. But the fact is, today's young people, no matter how sheltered, encounter a regular dose of sexually charged entertainment media messages.

So when do they hear the truth?

The world is full of explicit lies. Sadly, very few people are telling our kids the explicit truth. But we need to. I need to. You need to. If we don't, our kids will look for the answer somewhere else.

Several months ago, I was invited to speak to a bunch of middle school students about sex at an event at a church in the Chicago suburbs. The event brought out hundreds of kids, but noticeably less than their weekly attendance.

"Where are the others?" I asked, curious about the deficit in attendance.

"Their parents didn't let them come," the youth pastor explained. "We sent a letter to every parent explaining exactly what we'll be talking about. We always have a bunch of parents who don't think their kids are ready for that conversation."

"Are they ready?" I asked candidly, curious about this youth pastor's opinion.

"Most of the ones who aren't allowed to come are the ones who have the most unanswered questions. Sadly, they'll go to Google for the answers."

I wonder what they'll find there.

More Than Just the Talk

I just finished writing a book to parents titled *More Than Just the Talk*, encouraging and equipping moms and dads to create a comfortable climate for continual conversations about sex. When Dr. Kevin Leman read that book, his comment was, "In a world full of explicit lies, today's kids need parents who aren't afraid to tell them the explicit truth. This book provides parents with the tools they need to have these candid and continual conversations."

In that book I encouraged parents and adult mentors to speak openly about what the Bible says about sex, answering some of the big questions like, "Why should I wait?" and "How far can I go?" When we put that book together for parents, we began to ask ourselves, "Why not give them a resource they can give directly to their kids as well?"

So we created this resource to help you communicate truth on the subject. This little book is a tool that will not only clearly present God's design for sex, but also help provide honest answers to some of those common, candid . . . and yes, even embarrassing . . . questions about sex. I've even included discussion questions at the end of each chapter to help young people talk about what they've read and process what they've learned.

Are you ready to engage in these conversations?

Start Here

Unanswered Questions

L et's try something," Justin suggested in a whisper.

Melanie paused, pulling back from his embrace skeptically. "Try what?"

Melanie and Justin had been dating for only a few months, and Justin hadn't wasted any time putting the pressure on for her to sleep with him. She had refused his first few advances, but eventually obliged. It seemed *expected*.

Melanie loved Justin. He made her feel noticed . . . *and pretty*.

But recently Justin had been sharing some bizarre ideas. Last week he even suggested that Melanie make out with her friend Tori and film it. A little "girl-on-girl" action, he called it. Tori was an attractive sophomore with a reputation. Apparently Tori had tried it all.

Melanie wasn't excited about these wild proposals, but she didn't want to lose Justin either.

Justin touched Melanie's cheek affectionately. "My dad's gone tonight. I just thought we'd watch something together."

Last time, Justin showed Melanie something he streamed online, something she knew she shouldn't be watching.

Justin took an uneasy sip from the bottle, wiped his lip, and handed it to Melanie. "Here. You've barely had any of this."

Melanie had grown to recognize this familiar display. Justin was trying to work it. The drinks, the nervous tone of voice, the subtle suggestions. Justin was a completely different person when he was in this mode.

Where was the fun Justin who made her laugh?

Melanie felt trapped. Alone.

Was this normal? Was this what girls had to do to keep a guy?

Melanie wanted answers; but honestly, who was she going to talk to about *this*?

Colin was eighteen years old when he got Stephanie pregnant. Now he's twenty-one, single, working full time, going to school at night . . . all while taking care of his two-year-old son.

Colin never fathomed his life would be like this when Stephanie invited him up to her dorm room. In fact, he frequently looks back at that night, reflecting on each decision he made, wishing he had a do-over.

At age eighteen Colin left for college excited to be truly free to make his own decisions for the first time in his life. His parents had tried their best, but Colin felt smothered growing up in that house. They never trusted him or allowed him to do anything. At times they wouldn't even let him go to certain youth group activities. "We don't know who's going to be there or what they're going to allow," his parents would say.

But now Colin was out on his own and free to make his own choices. He liked his campus, enjoyed many of his professors, and made friends quickly. It was only about two months into school when he met Stephanie at a dance club.

"It's just what college guys do," Colin told me. "You go to the club on Friday night and you look for hot girls. It's what every song we listened to growing up told us to do. I guess I believed it."

Colin continued, "A friend introduced me to Stephanie and we danced together most of the night. We danced, kissed, hung out . . . and kissed some more. Next thing I knew we were in the car heading back to our dorms. She asked me if I wanted to come up to her room."

Colin was a virgin at the time.

"Didn't you know what might happen when you went up to her room?" I asked candidly.

"I don't know. I was just excited that she was into me. I mean, it's what every guy wants," Colin admitted. "I never really thought through if we'd *do it* that night, but next thing I knew we were on her bed alone and it was impossible to stop. It was like everything in our bodies was saying *yes*. The word *no* was the last thing on my mind."

"Had you ever talked with anyone about sex?" I asked.

"My dad talked to me about it once. He walked into my room awkwardly and asked me if I knew about sex. I told him I did. He said, 'Good. And you know you're supposed to wait until marriage, right?' I told him yes." Colin laughed. "And that was it. Everything a boy needs to know about sex."

No one had ever talked with Colin about this kind of temptation. Most of what he'd learned about sex was from *Two and a Half Men*.

⬛ ⬛ ⬛

Aaron's mom was browsing the family computer in search of a website she had visited recently. Instead, she found where her sixteen-year-old son had been browsing the night prior. As she saw the images unfold on the screen before her eyes, she literally burst into tears. She had never seen such perversion before. She could only ask one question.

"*Why?*"

Aaron told me when he arrived home that night his parents were both waiting up for him. "When I saw them both sitting there together on the couch with the TV off, I knew it was serious."

"My mom was bawling. She just kept asking me, 'Why?'"

"I couldn't tell her why," Aaron explained. "The only answer I could muster was, 'I don't know, but I just can't stop.'"

Aaron had wanted to tell someone, but who? What was he supposed to say? So he kept quiet for over a year.

Eventually his porn addiction revealed itself.

It always does.

If only Aaron had had someone to talk with . . .

Looking for Answers

Our culture creates a lot of confusion about sex. Honestly, sometimes it's difficult to know who's telling the truth.

On one hand, when we read our Bibles or go to church, we hear how God's design is to wait for sex and save that kind of intimacy for marriage. But on the other hand, when we go to school, turn on the TV, or listen to many of the songs on our favorite playlists . . . *they say quite the opposite.* Naturally, this makes many of us wonder.

Who's right?

Sex seems fun. How can something so natural be off-limits?

Many of us have questions. In the last two decades hanging out with teenagers I've heard them all:

Is hooking up really wrong?

What about living together once we fall in love? Everyone's doing it; isn't "waiting for marriage" a little outdated? Is it possible the whole concept of marriage is outdated?

If I believe in the Bible, what sex acts are specifically right or wrong before marriage? If the Bible just bans sex before marriage, is everything else fair game?

How about oral sex? Isn't that okay since it's not truly sex?

And . . . speaking truthfully, what about porn and masturbation? Why would God make something so fun, enticing, and pleasurable and then ban it from us? How cruel is that?

What about same-sex relationships? Since when does God deny any kind of true love?

Are you curious about the answers?

I was too. These are some of the same questions I had when I was a teenager . . . questions no one ever answered for me. That's why I'm going to answer all these questions in the pages of this little book.

My Questions

Let me be the first to tell you that my past isn't close to perfect in the area of sex and dating. I left a trail of hurt behind me in high school and college. I still look back in regret for some of the things I did—the consequences are still there.

I wish I had known then what I know now. I wish I had known the truth.

I'm not making excuses; I sincerely wish someone had answered my specific questions about sex when I was a teenager. Oh, sure, my parents told me all about the birds and the bees when I was growing up. And my dad probably would have answered my questions . . . *had I asked him.*

But I didn't ask. So questions remained.

Sure I took sex education in school. We learned all about the sperm swimming down the birth canal and fighting other sperm to get to that egg. The teacher (I believe he was also the driving instructor) taught us the official names of all the body parts. I was always just wishing he would show more pictures.

We learned about all those diseases—STDs. We saw pictures of open sores called chancres and venereal warts (not quite what I had in mind for pictures). But my questions were far from answered.

I went to church at the time and I remember my youth pastor talking about sex. He said sex was wrong before marriage and he always used that word I hated . . . *petting.* I don't like using a word that describes what I do to my dog for something sexual.

So . . . questions remained.

No one ever explained to me exactly what the Bible said about sex. I was pretty sure that it was wrong before marriage, but I couldn't really name the verse—and besides—it was just talking about intercourse, right? So I could do everything else? Second and third base were fair game . . . right?

I wanted answers.

Well . . . as long as they didn't mess up my fun.

I read about sex in every article, book, or magazine I could get my hands on looking for answers. Was I just curious? I can honestly say I wanted to know the truth, but at the same time, I was pretty happy rounding the bases as long as I avoided home plate. I knew in my heart this was wrong, but no one dared to reveal the explicit details about God's design for sex, even though the Bible is full of explicit details.

As I look back on my life, I have no greater regrets than how I behaved sexually before I was married. If I could change one thing about my past, I would remain sexually pure before marriage.

I'm not making excuses, but I really wish someone would have clearly communicated three facts I never understood:

1. Sex is good, and God gave it to us to enjoy. It's not bad or evil; it's not something to be ashamed of; it's an amazing gift given for you to enjoy with someone you don't intend to leave *ever* . . . your spouse. It's better than any hookup you can imagine.

2. This amazing gift of sexual intimacy is more than just "going all the way"; it's a passionate journey that begins with intimate touch, climaxes when two people have sexual intercourse, and includes everything in between.

3. Pornography and sexually charged entertainment media provoke lust, and lusting is the same as cheating on our spouse someday. Like it or not, that's adultery. Adultery is a big deal. We need to flee any temptations that cause us to lust or engage in sexual immorality.

I wish I had known these three facts, but I didn't. Sure, I had heard pieces of these truths, but no one ever told me in language I could understand. Nobody answered all my questions.

I never understood *sex matters*.

Who Has Answers?

Fast-forward to today and the situation is far scarier. Today, the world abounds in lies. Most of us have easy access to ginormous amounts of misinformation gushing through every screen, usually from advertisers or entertainers who are willing to show us and promise us anything . . . *for a price*. Are these really where the answers lie?

What is the truth?

Is sex really worth waiting for?

Is it actually feasible to refrain from sexual intimacy until marriage?

Could porn be a worthy pastime until we meet the right person . . . or is it harmful . . . or wrong?

What's right?

What's best?

What makes the most sense?

Great questions! Let's dive in and answer all of the above.

{1}

Why Wait?

Chris and Megan had each said they were going to wait until marriage for sex, but as their relationship progressed, they slowly began to question that notion.

By the time the two of them began their senior year of high school they had already been dating for seven months. What began as just holding hands and kissing early in the relationship quickly advanced to the next level.

Things seemed to get most passionate when the two of them were alone. Sometimes they would drive somewhere, park, and just start making out in the front seat of Chris's truck. Other times they'd be alone in Megan's room while her parents were downstairs making dinner. Regardless of the location, kissing led to touching, and as months passed, the touching became more intimate.

One day while Chris's parents were still at work, he and Megan lay on the couch in his basement watching TV. At first

Megan was just lying back against Chris as they watched a show together, but soon he began kissing her neck and touching her belly softly with his hands. It wasn't long before things heated up and shortly the two were passionately kissing, pressed up against each other. It had become almost routine.

But then Chris began to slide Megan's pants off.

"What are you doing?" she asked. Chris had never actually tried to undress her before.

He kissed her ear softly. "I don't know. I just want all of you."

Megan paused. "But isn't it wrong if we . . . you know . . . *do it?*"

He didn't stop. "Who really knows?" He looked into Megan's deep brown eyes. "Just do what feels right."

Megan had a difficult time coming up with a response. It *did* feel right. She loved Chris. Why not *make love?* It's not like many people were waiting for marriage anymore.

So why wait?

Chris and Megan aren't alone. Young people everywhere are wrestling with the question, "When is sex okay?" Some people seem to wait for marriage. Some wait until they're in love. Others just do it whenever they feel like it. *Who cares! It's fun.*

Is there a right answer? Or should we just go with what feels right at the moment?

Why Wait?

"Why wait?" It's the question I hear over and over again from countless young people today.

The question is probably a little more emphatic than that. If some teenagers said what they were truly thinking, it might sound more like this:

People engage in casual sexual activity in every TV show I watch and in every movie I enjoy. Whenever I am online, distracting pictures bombard me, begging me to click and see more, and honestly, I'm curious. Kids at school talk about sex, and my favorite songs obsess about it. Let's be real . . . everybody seems to think the idea of waiting is absurd!

But yet, my mom and dad tell me the Bible says to wait. Can I believe the Bible?

Give me just one compelling reason to wait! And don't try to scare me with teen pregnancy, because there are literally hundreds of kids doing it at my school and none of them . . . seriously, not one . . . is pregnant. (Okay, maybe one, but I really didn't know her that well, and she doesn't go to our school anymore anyway.)

There it is. Let's be honest. We're in the minority if we think sex is a gift to be enjoyed between married couples. We hear the opposite message every day.

Some of us might even be sorting it out in our own minds, weighing the evidence on both sides. "Should I really wait?" Have you ever heard a compelling answer to that question?

Have you ever heard the truth?

When I was a kid, I heard plenty of people tell me, "Wait until marriage for sex." But for me, I wanted to know why. *Why?* was huge. *Why* should I wait? I wanted to know all the facts so I could make my *own* decision.

Most of us aren't going to be convinced with "because the Bible says so." Some will want to see those passages for themselves. *Are they clear? Are you sure you didn't interpret them wrong?* Others might not even care what the Bible says. What then?

These are good questions. Interestingly enough, whether you care about the Bible or not, both research and common sense actually support what the Bible communicates clearly. In fact, I think the more you look at God's amazing gift of sex, the more you're going to see that God isn't trying to keep anything from you, He just wants a better life for you.

Let's take a look at three compelling reasons why waiting is wise. We won't just look at what the Bible says. In fact, we'll look at the answer scientifically, biblically, and logically.

⚠️ EXPLICIT WARNING:

In order to answer the question "Why wait?" adequately, I don't want to just provide you with a lame answer like, "Because it's smart!" or "Because the Bible says so." I'm guessing you want specifics. The following pages provide you with unedited specifics explaining the explicit truth about sexual satisfaction. Some of these specifics can get pretty detailed, but hang with it and you'll observe numerous compelling reasons why waiting is wise.

Let's start with scientific research.

1. The Scientific Answer

I spend quite a bit of time researching youth culture, attitudes, trends, and teen health. In any given week, I'll probably read a dozen articles and a handful of scientific studies about teenagers.

In the last two decades I've always paid particularly close attention to any studies about teen and adult sexuality, sexual satisfaction, and STDs. I speak to teenagers frequently and I always want to have the most current information.

STDs

Here's where many of you are expecting me to list all the STDs you could get if you engage in sexual activity. And that wouldn't be a bad approach, because one in four teenage girls in the U.S. has an STD.[1] Think about that for a second. That means if the girls in your school were a perfect cross section of all American teenage girls, out of 400 girls, 100 of them have an STD. Kind of scary.

The most common STD is HPV, the human papillomavirus, which is the number one leading cause of cervical cancer in women.[2] This disease is passed from person to person through any genital contact. People can get this even when using a condom, because condoms don't cover everything.[3] *You don't see that on a Trojan commercial.*

Chlamydia is another common STD, and it's a stealthy little sucker because it's asymptomatic. Male carriers rarely have any symptoms, so they just pass it on from person to person. Females usually don't feel the symptoms either, but the disease still does its work on them. By the time many girls discover they have it, they've got a pelvic inflammatory infection, a common culprit causing infertility in women. In short, they didn't know they had an STD, and now they can't have a baby someday.[4]

The list of STDs is long. I haven't even talked about the rampant spread of AIDS or herpes, both monsters with no cure. But instead of listing over twenty STDs and their consequences, let's take a peek at something else that research reveals about sex: *enjoyment.*

Monogamy Is More Enjoyable

Let's face it, people have sex because it's enjoyable. So let's look at *the most enjoyable sex.*

In writing this book I dove headfirst into a pile of recent studies from different perspectives. After reading through countless reports, I couldn't help but come to this conclusion: Monogamy is more enjoyable.

Let me give you a quick glimpse and you can make a decision for yourself.

Monogamy is a word I encounter quite a bit in research about sex and sexual satisfaction. *Monogamy* means "one partner." I am tempted to use the word *marriage* here, but the word *monogamy* doesn't always mean marriage. In today's world, it can also mean cohabitating couples who are "committed" to each other.

I'll leave it up to you to decide what you think the word *committed* truly means. Because when couples live together, they aren't committed enough to tie the knot in marriage, but they are saying, "I choose you . . . *for now.*"

That's the thing about today's "monogamous" relationships outside of marriage. They don't often stay true to the "mono" part of monogamy. When an unmarried "monogamous" man breaks it off with his partner and then begins living with a new woman, officially that is called "serial monogamy," which is monogamy with different people, but always one at a time. True monogamy is *one partner for life.* (Dare I say "marriage"?)

Research not only reveals the benefits of true monogamy, but also how much better *one partner for life* is compared to those with multiple partners past (serial monogamy) and multiple partners present (known as polygamy or polyamory) or promiscuity (sleeping with whoever I want whenever I want).

The bottom line is this: Most research points to the fact that sex is best saved for the intimacy of a true monogamous relationship, *one person for life.*

Here's a peek at some of the research on the subject.

A few years ago two sociologists did some research on the subject and wrote an entire book about it, *Premarital Sex in*

America. Their study looked at the sexual behaviors of today's young adults, and their findings weren't surprising.

As they compared monogamous couples (one partner) to individuals who were promiscuous (slept with whoever they wanted), they started to notice patterns. They discovered a significant correlation between the following:

- sexual restraint (the ability to say no) and emotional well-being
- monogamy and happiness
- promiscuity and depression

In fact, the happiest women they studied "were those with a current sexual partner and only one or two partners in their lifetime." And sadly, "a young woman's likelihood of depression rose steadily as her number of partners climbed and the present stability of her sex life diminished."[5] In other words, the more a woman slept around, the more depressed she became and her sex life grew worse.

Sexual Satisfaction

This research isn't unique. The more you look at unbiased studies, the more you'll discover people reported greater sexual satisfaction in monogamous relationships. In fact, this is nothing new.

Let's take a step back a few decades. In the early '90s a group of social scientists wrote a 718-page paper reporting the sexual habits of a large cross section of Americans. Several factors came as a surprise to many.

First, the report found there was more emotional satisfaction and physical pleasure for those in a monogamous relationship than for those who had sexual relations with one or more other partners within the past twelve months. In fact, in a sample of 868 women located in fifteen states, the women with many partners expressed the least sexual satisfaction. The more people they slept with, the less happy they were with sex.[6]

Second, the report found a direct correlation between "religious belief" and sexual pleasure. In fact, the study found that the people who have the most sex, experience the best sex, and are the happiest with their sex lives are monogamous, married, religious people. The religious people actually reported more orgasms:

> Women without religious affiliation were the least likely to report always having an orgasm with their primary partner— only one in five. . . . Protestant women who reported always having an orgasm was the highest, at nearly one-third. In general, having a religious affiliation was associated with higher rates of orgasm for women (27 percent of both Catholic and Type I Protestants reported always having an orgasm with their primary partner.)[7]

The authors couldn't help but conclude, "Religion may be independently associated with rates of orgasm."[8]

Whodathunkit?

This wasn't the first study to find the correlation between religion and sexual satisfaction. In fact, one of the largest studies ever attempted found the same thing. *Redbook* magazine surveyed over 100,000 women in the early '70s. They found monogamous women to be more sexually satisfied, and those who went to church even more so.[9]

It didn't matter if the reports were from last year or the last century, I kept reading the same thing—monogamous couples using terms like *sexual satisfaction* and *happiness*. In fact, some use the word *happiness* in the title of their studies, like a recent report by two economists entitled *Money, Sex, and Happiness*.

This paper even used the word *marriage*, labeling those in monogamous, faithful marriages the happiest. They found those who cheated on their spouses "less happy" and those who paid for sex "much less happy" than others.[10]

But let's be honest. Are all the reports saying this? Even the recent ones? Because if you're like me, you've stood in line at the grocery store and seen titles of articles on the magazine racks like "How an Affair Will Boost Your Marriage."

Is this true? Are people who have affairs happier in the long run?

To answer that question, let's look at this word we keep seeing over and over again: *happiness*.

Defining "Happiness"

Most of the reports above seem to use words like *happiness* or *sexual satisfaction*. What does that really mean?

Mark White, Ph.D., offers some good insight into perceived happiness in a recent *Psychology Today* article. He starts off the article declaring "It doesn't take much to see that monogamy and promiscuity can each give a person happiness, albeit likely two different kinds."

In other words, Dr. White is saying that both monogamy and promiscuity can make someone "happy." But each produces a different kind of happy.

Take a look at what he discovered and determine which kind of "happiness" you want.

Promiscuity—The Thrill of the Moment

Promiscuity, or "nonmonogamy" as he calls it, "brings the excitement of variety, the thrill of the unknown, and the pure physical bliss of sex, untethered by any emotional attachment or anxiety."

Monogamy—Longer-Lasting Fulfillment

On the other hand, monogamy provides "a deeper, longer-lasting, and more fulfilling type of happiness that enhances any other aspects of one's life."

I can't say I disagree with his premise. It's almost like he's saying, "Sin is fun for the moment." His observation basically surmises that if we go around having sex with anyone we want, we're going to experience the "bliss" and pleasure that sex brings, without the hassle of emotional attachment, for those who find it a hassle. We'd be fools to deny the temporary and quick thrill of sin. If it wasn't fun, we probably wouldn't do it.

Sin can be fun . . . *for the moment.*

The question is . . . what about the next morning?

What about hurt feelings?

What about unwanted pregnancy?

What about sexually transmitted diseases?

What about guilt, shame, or regret?

White says, "The ideal would be to find the more hedonic, animalistic pleasure with his or her spouse or partner instead of looking for it outside the marriage or relationship." I can't help but agree!

So what are you truly looking for? Are you looking for the quick thrill or, to use White's words, "the longer-lasting and more fulfilling type of happiness"?[11]

For the last twenty years as a minister, I've not only worked with youth and young adults, I've counseled young couples, performed a handful of marriages, and acted as a lay leader for a young-couples class and a class for parents of teenagers. In all my years dialoguing with young couples, I've never, not even once, heard one of them say, "I'm so glad that I slept around when I was younger!"

Quite the contrary, actually. Couples with promiscuous pasts often have to work through issues of jealousy, comparison, and other forms of hurt that arise.

Rarely will you find a nonmonogamous relationship where there is peace. Usually someone is feeling left out and the issues of pain and hurt overflow. Sure, some marriages need work too. But those problems greatly increase when you add other partners into the mix.

It's almost like the human heart just wasn't created for multiple partners.

God created us to enjoy sex in a relationship where we'll never need to worry about disease, never need to compare with others, and never feel guilty afterward. Those who have sex in marriage enjoy a longer-lasting, more fulfilled happiness and are more satisfied with sexual intimacy with their spouse.

God wants us to enjoy the most enjoyable sex, and that's in marriage. In fact . . . it was his plan from the beginning. Let's look at the place where this is documented.

2. The Biblical Answer

Why should you wait until marriage to have sex?

That's the big question we're seeking to answer here. And the Bible provides a great answer:

Because God Created Sex for Us to Enjoy in Marriage for Life.

As we discussed in the previous section, God's design is ultimately the most enjoyable. And the Bible confirms it! Does that surprise you?

When many of us think of the Bible we think of the "thou shalt not" passages. Perhaps we should take a peek at what the Bible is telling us to enjoy instead.

I promised I'd tell you the explicit truth, and the plain, un-diluted truth is that God created sex to *enjoy* in *marriage* for life. In order to show you this, let's look at two words: *enjoy* and *marriage*.

ENJOY

God's design for sex is evident all through the Bible, and the closer you look, the more you'll see how awesome a gift sex is for us to enjoy. Start from the beginning of the Bible . . . *the very beginning* . . . like the book of Genesis.

The Bible opens with the story of a naked man named Adam in a garden. As Adam walked around and looked at all the animals, he was lonely and wanted a companion more like him.

God noticed this. In Genesis 2:18, God said, "It is not good for the man to be alone."

So what did God do?

Poof. A naked woman!

Seriously. God makes a naked woman for the naked man. It's right there in the Bible in Genesis 2. (God is so cool!)

It gets better. Once God made them both, he told them, "Be fruitful and multiply" (Genesis 1:28). How's that for a sexual green light?

My guess is that God probably didn't even need to convince them to do this.

Some people miss God's awesome gift of sexual enjoyment here because they assume that God's command to "be fruitful and multiply" just meant "have babies." But God's creation was so much more than this. Why did God give both man and woman pleasure centers on their genitals? Think about that for a second. Do you know that a woman's clitoris has no purpose whatsoever other than to provide sexual pleasure? The pleasure centers on the head of the penis are the same way. God gave us the awesome gift of sex for us to *enjoy*.

If you're a parent and you are screening this book first to see if it's acceptable for your kid, I encourage you not to let this fact frighten you. The Bible isn't afraid to talk about sex because it's revealed as a gift for us to *enjoy* in *marriage* (and we'll talk about that marriage part very soon). The Bible tells us the unedited truth throughout its pages.

Sex isn't naughty. In fact, God is a big advocate for sex when you find that person and commit to him or her in marriage. Take Proverbs 5:18–19, for example:

> Let your wife be a fountain of blessing for you.
> Rejoice in the wife of your youth.
> She is a loving deer, a graceful doe.
> Let her breasts satisfy you always.
> May you always be captivated by her love.

Many young people don't even know the Bible talks like this. But the plain, unedited truth is that God wants a husband to *enjoy* his wife's breasts. The Bible isn't afraid to say that explicitly. (We'll actually look a little bit deeper into this passage in chapter 4 when we talk about the lure of pornography.)

LONG-TERM FULFILLMENT

Sex is very pleasurable. Just looking at his wife's body can be a stimulating experience for a husband. God made it that way. But let me be clear. God's creation of sexual enjoyment goes much beyond immediate pleasure. God actually also provides a long-term fulfillment for two people to share when they join together as one (Genesis 2:24) and live as partners for life.

Sex is a big part of this union as "one." It's a special gift created for married couples to share uniquely, and their relationship actually becomes more connected the more the two of them are intimate with each other.

The human body releases a powerful hormone called oxytocin when you hug or kiss someone you really care about. This hormone, often called the bonding hormone, or cuddle hormone, is stimulated big time during sex. It actually deepens the feelings of attachment each time a couple has sex. In one study, men were given oxytocin while they looked at pictures of women—including complete strangers, women they were acquainted with, and women they were in love with. The pleasure and desire regions of their brains lit up at the mere sight of the women they loved.[12]

This is why the pain of a breakup is so great. Think of the thousands of songs written about this kind of hurt. The more we bond with someone and share the most intimate part of ourselves . . . the more it rips us apart when we separate.

It's almost as if the creator behind the design of all this didn't want us to make that sexual connection unless we meant to stay together, eh?

Marriage

But some people try to get the sexual enjoyment without having to commit to the obligation of marriage.

It makes sense. People like the immediate pleasure sex provides—so much so that they wonder if they can enjoy that quick thrill with lots of partners. They might see marriage as a hassle, not a long-term fulfillment, so they seek the pleasure of a one-night stand or even sex with a prostitute.

God knew people would do this so he addressed this explicitly in Scripture. In fact, there are warnings in the Bible about sex for married people, single people, and even people who think it might be okay for them to just think about sex. Yes, these warnings are the "thou shalt not" passages.

What About Sex With People Other Than My Spouse?

Sadly, people often try to do things their own way rather than the way God intended. They think, *Sex is fun, so I'll have it with others as well, not just my spouse.* We see numerous examples of people trying this all through the Bible, even in the first book: Judah (Genesis 38), the people of Sodom and Gomorrah (Genesis 19), and many of the Israelites.

So God warned them in the Ten Commandments, in Exodus 20:14: "You must not commit adultery." That's pretty clear. It means don't have sex outside of marriage.

Again, this isn't because sex was bad or because God wanted to deny their fun. Quite the contrary. He actually created an amazing plan where one man and one woman could join together in a unique bond for the rest of their lives, committed to each other and enjoying the pleasure of sexual intimacy, something the two of them would share exclusively.

So stick with your spouse. If you go outside of the marriage relationship for sex, there are consequences. (Research revealed this to us a few pages back.)

What About Sex If I'm Not Married Yet?

Some people might ask, "Well, I'm not married. Isn't it okay to have sex, because I won't be cheating on my spouse . . . since I don't have a spouse?"

First, you have to question the logic there. Just because you don't have a husband or wife yet doesn't mean that you should go bonding with a bunch of other people now. Think of what we know so far about this process. God wants us to enjoy sex with one person for life. That doesn't license us to sleep with a bunch of people before we're married. Everything we do before marriage will be carried into the marriage relationship.

Just in case you missed that logic, the apostle Paul addresses this throughout the New Testament, like in this passage: "Run from sexual sin! No other sin so clearly affects the body as this one does. For sexual immorality is a sin against your own body" (1 Corinthians 6:18).

You'll notice that verse uses the term *sexual sin*. Most translations of the Bible will use the words *sexual sin* or *sexual immorality* here. Older translations use the word *fornication*. They all mean the same thing: "the voluntary sex of an unmarried person." I say *voluntary* because it means the person has a choice. Sadly, many young people have been abused or raped. That victim didn't sin. But if you have the choice, and you choose to have sex before you're married, that is "sexual sin." (For those who are curious, the original Greek word here is *porneia* or *pornos*, which are the root words for the English words *pornography* or *pornographic*. If your pastor looks it up in his Greek dictionary, it will say something like "the surrendering of sexual purity; promiscuity of any or every type.")

In other words, run from any temptation to have sex with someone if you're not married to them. Paul uses this term again in Ephesians 5:3: "Let there be no sexual immorality, impurity, or greed among you. Such sins have no place among God's people."

I like the way the New International Version of the Bible words this verse: "There must not be even a hint of sexual immorality" among you. It's pretty clear. Don't have sex outside of the marriage relationship.

And just in case we've missed either of these categories, Hebrews 13:4 addresses both adulterers and fornicators (both married people and unmarried people who want to have sex with others): "Marriage should be honored by all, and the marriage bed kept pure, for God will judge the adulterer and all the sexually immoral" (Hebrews 13:4 NIV).

It seems pretty crystal clear, right?

What About Just Thinking About Sex?

Well, some people still try to find a loophole. Maybe porn is okay, right? Because then we aren't actually having sex with anyone else. We're just sort of . . . *pretending to have sex*!

During the time Jesus was walking around on earth he encountered some people like this. They were thinking, *So as long as I don't have sex, it's okay. I'll just think about it in my mind!*

Jesus himself decided to address this, calling it *lust* and labeling it just as bad as adultery.

> You have heard the commandment that says, "You must not commit adultery." But I say, anyone who even looks at a woman with lust has already committed adultery with her in his heart. So if your eye—even your good eye—causes you to lust, gouge it out and throw it away. It is better for you to lose one part of your body than for your whole body to be thrown into hell.
>
> Matthew 5:27–29

Jesus wasn't pulling any punches here.

If you're thinking about it, you're no better than someone who is doing it.

And if you have any doubts about how serious Jesus was about this, just read that part about plucking your eye out again.

God's Design Makes Sense

God's plan for sex was simple: one man, one woman, committing to each other in marriage and enjoying sexual intimacy for life. Anything outside of that plan was not only forbidden, it caused problems. It ripped lives apart.

It's funny how you see the truth of God's creation even in pop entertainment. You'll watch an episode of a popular show like *New Girl*, where two main characters seek to "hook up" with someone in search of meaningless sex. Eventually, after sleeping together for a while, you see them begin to bond . . . and they are surprised by this. In addition, if they break up, they are hurt and wonder why.

Maybe because God made it that way?

Yes . . . God's design just makes sense. So let's take a moment and answer the question "Why wait?" logically.

3. The Logical Answer

Close your eyes and picture the world for a minute. Picture it exactly how you see it every day. Picture the things you find beautiful and the things you enjoy, what makes you laugh, what makes you smile. But let's be realistic. Let's also recognize some of the pain in this world: wars, world hunger, sickness, brutality, death . . . the list goes on. This is the world we live in.

Now I want you to make one small adjustment to this image, one little tweak to change your picture. Just imagine the world exactly like it is now . . . but with one exception: Pretend that, for some reason, everyone in the entire world believes God's plan for sex and marriage and stays true to their one spouse for life.

The world still has suicide, crime, high-school dropouts, and all other kinds of pain and hurt. If you ride your bike to the grocery store and leave it out front unlocked, it will be gone within five minutes because people steal things in this world.

But even with all this pain and hurt, for some unknown reason, imagine this one little change: Every single person believes God's plan to wait until marriage for sex, and no one performs any sexual activity outside of the marriage relationship. No one lusts after one another, and once they get married they love each other and stay committed to their spouse, enjoying a sexual intimacy with just the two of them for the rest of their lives.

Picture this world:

- For starters, in this world Dad doesn't trade in his wife for a younger version.
- This is a world with no dads cheating on moms, or moms cheating on dads.
- There are no painful family splits because couples actually love each other and stay committed to each other in this world.
- This is a world with no pornography, because no one is lusting and no one would pose for sexual pictures for that purpose.
- This is a world with no prostitution, because sex is only for marriage.
- This is a world with no pedophiles (people who sexually abuse children), no molestation, and no sexual abuse of any kind, because again, sex is only between a husband and wife in the intimacy of marriage.
- This world doesn't have any *Who's Your Daddy?* reality TV shows.
- This is a world with no STDs. No AIDS would be transmitted sexually, no gonorrhea, no herpes, no syphilis.
- This is a world with no chlamydia, the asymptomatic STD that often leads to pelvic inflammatory disease and eventually infertility problems in women.
- This is a world with no HPV, the human papillomavirus, which is the leading cause of cervical cancer in women.[13]
- This is a world with very few abortions, because 83 percent of abortions are performed *on women who are not married.*[14]
- This is a world with no rape.
- This is a world with no sex slavery.

. . . the list goes on. All this if people just trusted God in this one area of their lives. Imagine if they trusted him in everything.

Let me ask you . . . does God's way sound so bad?

Bottom Line

Sex is worth the wait.

I got married at twenty years old. I've now been married over twenty years. It's weird looking back . . . I actually have lived more years married than I have single.

God's gift of marriage is such an amazing blessing. My wife, Lori, and I are friends, we're kayaking buddies, we run together, we eat at Buffalo Wild Wings together, and also at the fancy fish place she likes . . .

. . . *and we're lovers.*

Someday, like Adam in the garden next to his naked wife, Eve, you will realize that the greatest thing that God ever invented is lying right next to you in your marriage bed. And you get to enjoy connecting with that person, in so many exciting ways, for the rest of your life.

God's design just makes sense. When we have sex outside of God's design, we bring consequences on ourselves: physical consequences, emotional consequences, and spiritual consequences. If we look at the outcome of our choices, it's even more evident that God's way is best.

God wants us to enjoy sex with the person we marry forever. He doesn't want us to have a sneak preview. It's wrong and it robs us of that special gift. God has given us the gift of sex to enjoy in marriage.

Treasure that gift . . . *the way God intended it.*

But that begs the question, "If I want to wait for sex until marriage, how far can I go sexually?" We'll answer that question in the next chapter . . .

Discussion Questions

1. In the opening to this chapter we read the story of Chris and Megan, who believed in waiting for sex until marriage yet found themselves questioning the truth of that notion as their relationship progressed. Finally, in the heat of the moment, Chris pronounced, "Just do what feels right." Why do you think their beliefs began changing as their relationship progressed?

2. How do we determine what is best for us sexually? Is there a good source of knowledge or authority that influences you in this decision? (Biblical instructions, scientific research, logical truths . . .)

3. Why do you think scientific research repeatedly shows promiscuous people (who sleep with whoever they want) are not only more sexually unsatisfied, but also more vulnerable to depression?

4. Why do you think research showed monogamous people (those with one partner) to be happier and more sexually satisfied?

5. Dr. Mark White defined two types of sexual "happiness": the animalistic thrill-of-the-moment happiness you can experience when you are promiscuous (sleeping with whoever you want) and a deeper, longer-lasting, more fulfilling happiness when you are monogamous (have one partner for life). Which one do you think sounds better in the long run? Can a monogamous person experience both the quick thrill of sex and the longer-lasting happiness?

6. What are some of the consequences we might encounter when we choose promiscuous activities?

7. How is the powerful hormone oxytocin evidence that people are designed to stay together?

8. Read the following passage of Scripture: "Run from sexual sin! No other sin so clearly affects the body as this one does. For sexual immorality is a sin against your own body" (1 Corinthians 6:18). This chapter gives a definition of the words *sexual immorality* (also translated as *fornication*) used in this verse. Explain that definition in your own words.

9. Why does Paul, the author of 1 Corinthians, warn people to flee or run from this kind of sin?

10. Your Christian friend is considering sleeping with his girlfriend and asks for your advice. Using one or more of the passages of Scripture in this chapter, what would you advise him?

11. When you imagined a world where everyone listens to God in one area—believing in his plan for love, sex, and marriage—what impacted you about this world?

12. What is something you read in this chapter that you can really use?

How Far?

During high school I had a serious girlfriend. We dated for almost a year and we spent every possible moment together. We started as friends, but that quickly escalated to something more.

I waited about a month to kiss her for the first time. I won't bore you with the details, but within a few months, our relationship grew more physical. It wasn't uncommon for our time together to include long make-out sessions.

Something began happening. The more time we spent just kissing and making out, the more difficult it was to stop it from progressing to something further.

If you have ever had a serious relationship, you probably know exactly what I'm talking about. It's almost as if God's design is that once you start passionately kissing . . . *you want to keep going*!

This is where the inevitable question is asked:

How far can we go?

It's the biggest question Christians in relationships are forced to wrestle with almost every day.

Some couples never discuss it. This is the surest way to fail. *Just hope it doesn't progress.* Any couple who has dated for any length of time and spends time alone will quickly discover that kissing leads to passionate embraces, which evolve to touching . . . until soon it would take a dad holding a shotgun to stop things from progressing further!

Those couples who do address the question usually are searching for a line. If they've read the Bible at all and studied some of the verses we've already addressed in this book, they know that sex is for marriage. But what is *sex*? Many think, *Sex is just intercourse, right?*

So the search for "the line" begins.

Some will allow touching above the waist, others allow touching below the waist. Some will even allow oral sex, because *it's not sex, right? Uh . . . even though it has the word* sex *in it.*

Some come up with a viable solution, rubbing against each other with clothes on. I think couples feel a little less guilty with this one because there is no actual touching of hands to skin. Although couples who allow this can actually bring each other to climax, even with clothes on.

Is this going too far?

Loopholes

When I was in high school I believed in the Bible and its message of "no sex until marriage." But to me everything else was fair game.

Oh, I didn't truly believe that. In all honesty, in the back of my mind I figured that oral sex was probably wrong, and I didn't even allow myself to consider the morality of any "below the waist" activity. So during those years I made sexual decisions using blurred lines and messy morality. I "kind of" knew some of it was wrong, but I definitely didn't know where the line was.

Whenever we talked about sex in youth group, I was curious. In hindsight, I think I was looking for a stamp of approval more than anything else. Like those Pharisees in the Bible, I wanted to see a list of do's and don'ts . . . *and look for a loophole.* I had a talent for finding loopholes. (I should have been a lawyer.)

I remember hearing sex talks where they told me that "petting" was bad. I can barely type that word without shuddering. Man, that word is awkward. But for some reason youth workers in the '80s would use the word to describe intimate touching below the waist. "Petting is wrong. Don't do it," they told us. But I never heard a good explanation for why, other than the chance that the girl's dad would find out and hunt me down (which is a pretty compelling reason, I might add).

So I remember walking away from these discussions thinking, *Okay, no hands touching below the waist.*

But rubbing up against each other with clothes on was fair game!

A loophole!

No one ever taught me the explicit truth. And yes, the Bible is very explicit on the subject.

So how can we discover the answer to the question, "How far can I go?"

Consider baseball.

Sex Is a Process

Sex isn't just intercourse. It starts way before that. Consider the proverbial baseball analogy.

"I got to third base with her."

You may have heard your friends using this age-old correlation. Of course there is no reference book. *The bases* were just explained to us on the playground some day when we were young.

First base is kissing.

Second base is touching above the waist.

Third base is touching below the waist (and probably includes oral sex in most circles).

A *home run is "going all the way," or "intercourse," to use the scientific term.*

Maybe we didn't hear about the bases all at once, but we've heard them referred to.

The analogy is actually pretty good, because in baseball you round the bases. You don't just run straight to third. A guy usually doesn't walk up to his girlfriend and just stick his hands down her pants. Nor does a husband with his wife. If so, he'd be slapped and called a pig.

We have an official term for rounding the bases: *foreplay.*

As you can see, sex isn't just intercourse. Sex is a process that starts with passionate kissing, progresses to embracing, touching . . . and eventually ends with intercourse.

Lovers never start with intercourse. It's impossible, really. The body doesn't work like that. A rapist goes straight to intercourse, and not only hurts a woman emotionally because of the lack of consent, but most often does all kinds of damage physically because her body wasn't ready for it.

So why all these graphic details?

Because it's important for us to understand sexuality and how the body works. Sex is a beautiful process that begins with foreplay and peaks at intercourse.

Why Is It So Difficult to Stop?

Any teen who has been alone with someone they are attracted to and allowed the process to start knows that it is like trying to stop a forest fire after a drought!

So why is it so difficult to stop?

Because it's not supposed to be stopped!

The truth is, God made this process so that when a husband sees his wife wearing something sexy, his motor starts running. They kiss and embrace. Soon, his pulse will accelerate, his penis will grow erect (keeping it in scientific terms), and her vagina will start to lubricate naturally. They might touch each other intimately, caressing various parts of the body, places no other person touches, places reserved for a husband and a wife. Eventually the man will insert his penis into the vagina, and the two will eagerly move in a motion that provides stimulation to both male and female until one or both climax.

The whole process is amazing and euphoric . . . and yes, a little awkward to talk about. After all, it is an intimate act designed for a husband and wife to share privately.

So why the human anatomy and sexuality lesson?

Because those who are asking, "How far can I go?" need to understand that this process is for marriage. The *entire process* is only for marriage.

I can hear it now. "*What? Are you saying kissing is only for marriage?*"

I've heard that question. I've heard it from teenagers who are just like I was at their age, teenagers who want to know the exact line so they can find a loophole. Some people seem to prefer a list of what you can and can't do.

THE LEGALIST'S LIST

Kissing—*yes*

Hugging—*yes*

Hand to fully clothed breasts—*no*

Hand to genitals—*no*

Big toe to kneecap—*as long as you are wearing socks*

Jumping rope—*sounds fun, so no*

This is ridiculous. Whenever we start making up lists of rules, we tend to look less like Jesus and more like the Pharisees. The Pharisees made huge lists and were still corrupt. So forget the list. Let me do one better. Let me teach you how to understand truth and make wise decisions based on good information.

The truth is, God wants us to share *this intimate process of sex* within marriage. We learned that in great detail in the last chapter. No one who has even a remedial understanding of Scripture would argue that. The argument always arises with "How far can I go?"

Don't Start the Process

I just proposed that unmarried couples shouldn't even begin the process.

"Prove it!" I would have declared when I was a teenager.

Okay. Exhibit A: *Jesus' teaching on lust.*

Remember this passage from the previous chapter? Jesus himself addressed lust, labeling it just as sinful as adultery.

> You have heard the commandment that says, "You must not commit adultery." But I say, anyone who even looks at a woman with lust has already committed adultery with her in his heart.
>
> Matthew 5:27–28

Or 2 Timothy 2:22, where Paul simply said, "Run from anything that stimulates youthful lusts."

Do you know any young man who can lie on top of his girlfriend, passionately kissing and groping her breasts (second base) . . . *and not lust?*

Seriously. What is going through this guy's mind at the moment? Is he thinking about feeding homeless people? Is he thinking about his math homework? Not a chance. His mind is 110 percent focused on her body and how much he wants it. Everything within him wants to go further.

It's hard to deny this kind of excitement, because the body will evidence it in so many ways. God designed it perfectly so. When a couple gets into an intimate situation, heartbeats quicken, adrenaline flows through the bloodstream, the penis hardens, and the vagina gets wet. The human bodies start preparing for one of the greatest physical pleasures imaginable, an intimate bond that a husband and wife can share uniquely together. Dopamine rushes through the brain, stimulating even greater pleasure, and oxytocin is secreted by the posterior pituitary gland, inspiring greater bonding.

The bodies get excited and begin this sexually intimate process that prepares them for intercourse. This whole process is a good thing when you are married. At the same time, this is something we shouldn't *initiate* before we're married.

I think of a classic show your parents probably watched years ago, *Everybody Loves Raymond*. In one episode Raymond was walking around in his boxers cleaning the house and his wife, Debra, came in the room, noticed him cleaning, and got turned on. (Yes, that is the key to a woman's heart. Get off your butt and do something around the house!) She walked up to him and began kissing him passionately.

Suddenly, they realized his parents were about to come over, so she stopped her sexual advance. Frustrated with Debra, Raymond exclaimed, "What are you doing to me here?! You can't kiss me like that. . . . You've activated the launch sequence!"

That's a great line, and in all honesty, it probably just answered the question we've been asking this entire chapter, "How far can we go?"

Don't "activate the launch sequence."

No, I'm *not* saying *you can't kiss*. Again, it's not about a list of do's and don'ts. In fact, I often word it the same way I worded it in my advice to guys in my rather candid book *The Guy's Guide to God, Girls and the Phone in Your Pocket:* "Don't do anything with your girlfriend you wouldn't do in front of your grandmother."

It's like this. Let's say you're a teenage guy and your family throws a big dinner for your birthday, inviting the entire extended family and your girlfriend. After dinner you open presents. Your girlfriend gives you a really nice gift and you lean over and give her a kiss in front of everyone. She blushes, the adults smile, and your little brother exclaims, "Ew, gross!"

Sounds innocent.

Now picture the exact same scenario, same crowd, same present from the girlfriend . . . but this time, when you lean over and kiss her, you start becoming a little more passionate. Instead of just kissing her, you crawl on top of her and start kissing her neck and breathing heavy.

Who would do this?

Chances are Dad might spray you with the garden hose!

Why wouldn't a teenage guy do this in front of Grandma and the whole family?

Perhaps because it's . . . *intimate?* And intimate situations like this usually progress to something else. The world teaches us, "Who cares if it progresses to something else?" But God's design is that intimate situations like this are really reserved for two people who have committed to each other for life in marriage.

The Wrong Question

I commonly hear young people ask, "How far is too far?" That's like asking me, "How close to the fire can I get without getting burnt?" Sadly, the only way to find out is to *get burnt.*

Newsflash: We don't have to learn everything the hard way.

So whenever a young couple asks me, "How far should we go?" I respond, "You're asking me the wrong question. The better question is, 'How far away can we stay?'"

Let's look at the situation. From what we've discussed so far, most of us have concluded a few things:

1. God's design is the best way—I want to wait until marriage for sex.

2. Sex isn't just intercourse—it's the whole process. After all, Jesus said lusting is the same as actually doing it. Paul told us to run from this kind of temptation.

3. I shouldn't even initiate the process until I'm married—because the process is meant to be finished. And there's only one person I want to start and finish the process with—my future spouse!

With these things in mind, maybe we should be asking, "How can I be successful in saving myself for my spouse?"

Sex is a huge temptation for us today—not just couples, but anyone:

- the twelve-year-old gamer sitting in front of the computer
- the twenty-one-year-old college student invited to go clubbing with her friends
- the sixteen-year-old high school fullback who is being encouraged by all his buddies to "get laid"
- the fifteen-year-old girlfriend who is feeling pressure from her boyfriend

The world is screaming, "Just do it." And our bodies aren't always disagreeing.

The biggest issue many of us are going to have to address is, *Do I want to live for the truth, and make godly choices, or live for the quick thrill of the moment?*

Those who want to stay pure need to realize the draw of sexual temptation and avoid it at all costs.

Maybe that's why the Bible often uses the word *flee*. But what does that actually look like? Let's dissect that in the next chapter.

Discussion Questions
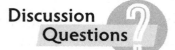

1. Several stories in this book reveal that the more time couples spent kissing and making out, the more difficult it was to stop from progressing to something further. Why is this common?

2. What are some of the lines or boundaries you have seen people set regarding how far they can go? Do you agree? Why or why not?

3. Foreplay includes passionate kissing, embracing, and eventually intimate touching. Quick biology quiz: What specifically happens to the male and female bodies during foreplay that prepares them for sex?

4. Why can't two people have instantaneous sex without foreplay?

5. Why did the author say it is very difficult to stop sex right in the middle of foreplay?

6. When does the "launch sequence" start for most males?

7. Read the following passage of Scripture:

> You have heard the commandment that says, "You must not commit adultery." But I say, anyone who even looks at a woman with lust has already committed adultery with her in his heart.
>
> Matthew 5:27–28

What is a good definition for lusting?

8. Can a guy touch a girl's breasts, even outside her shirt, without lusting? Explain (and if you said yes, then please explain what he's possibly thinking about when he does this . . . and if said guy has a pulse).

9. Why is "How far can I go?" the wrong question?

10. Summarizing what you read in this chapter, and from the Scriptures provided, how far is too far?

Fleeing

Fact: Dentists have recommended that a toothbrush be kept at least six feet away from a toilet to avoid airborne particles resulting from the flush.

How many of you are going to store your toothbrush just five feet away? It's only a foot closer than the dentist recommends. Maybe only a few urine particles will splash on your toothbrush.

How many of you are going to store it right next to the toilet by the toilet paper roll? You could build a little shelf right there.

How many of you want to hang it by a string in the toilet bowl so that it is practically rinsed every time you flush?

The thing about the subject of sexual temptation that always amuses me is the amount of risk people are willing to take. Actually, using the word *risk* isn't accurate. The thing about this subject that always surprises me is how *stupid* we are willing to be just to fulfill an urge.

Sadly, people often leave their brains at home when they embark on sexual decisions. It's foolish to wait until we're in a

57

sexual situation to decide what we're going to do. Almost any person is going to choose sex when *in the situation*. It's the way God wired us. It's what we're programmed to do.

I'll proceed cautiously because I know I'm about to step on sacred territory. But the fact is that many of us allow sexual messages and imagery into our lives daily through our technology and our entertainment media sources. And before you have a chance to say, "Oh, those lyrics and images don't affect me," let's just take a quick peek at what the experts say.

The journal *Pediatrics* released a study a few years ago revealing the obvious: "Teens whose iPods are full of music with raunchy, sexual lyrics start having sex sooner than those who prefer other songs." The study was very specific:

> Teens who said they listened to lots of music with degrading sexual messages were almost twice as likely to start having intercourse or other sexual activities within the following two years as were teens who listened to little or no sexually degrading music. Among heavy listeners, 51 percent started having sex within two years, versus 29 percent of those who said they listened to little or no sexually degrading music.[1]

Sexual imagery has a similar effect. A recent study in the journal *Psychological Science* revealed that promiscuous programming promotes real-life promiscuity. In other words, if we watch people hooking up on our screens, the chances are higher we will hook up in real life. In fact:

> Young teens who viewed movies with sexual content were profoundly influenced by what they watched. They initiated sexual behavior earlier than their peers who had viewed less sexual content, and they tended to imitate the on-screen sexual behaviors they saw—which included casual sex, having multiple partners and high-risk behaviors.[2]

Forget these experts for a second and let me ask you an honest question. Are you fleeing sexual temptation when you are watching or listening to sexually charged entertainment?

Perhaps we should listen to the Bible's advice and flee sexual immorality and lustful pleasures. Let's look at what this looks like for each gender.

A Word for the Girls—What Fleeing Looks Like (Guys, You Can Peek at This Too)

When most people think of the need to flee, they probably think of males. After all, more males look at porn, more males admit to masturbating, and males seem to have a much stronger sex drive than females.

Yes, girls might not be just like boys, but it doesn't mean they don't have a sex drive. God happened to make sex very pleasurable, not to mention a natural desire when you love someone. So girls can be vulnerable to sexual temptation, just like boys. But more commonly, girls give sex to get love.

It's sad but true. It's like this:

Guys give love to get sex.

Girls give sex to get love.

Stop and read those above statements one more time.

Again, this isn't to say that girls don't enjoy sex. Girls often enjoy consensual sex on several levels. But frequently, girls are giving sex because they know that it's what guys want, and from day one, they have been taught that being sexy is an important part of being a woman. The American Psychological Association calls this "the sexualization of girls."[3] It's when girls feel that their value comes from being sexy rather than other characteristics. Subconsciously, sex fills a need of acceptance.

"He wants me. That means he likes me and values me."

If only.

When females engage in sexually intimate situations they not only feel valued, they often feel the natural pleasure that goes along with sexual activity. Sex triggers dopamine releases, which feels good, and oxytocin, which makes you feel closer to someone. So it's hard to deny the draw of sex for anyone, male or female.

Just like males, females can be susceptible to sexual temptation and need to take the Bible's advice to "flee." Girls need to understand why sex is worth the wait (as we discussed in chapter 1) and how to avoid "starting the launch sequence."

What does this look like for teenage girls today?

1. Understand How Guys Think

Girls sometimes assume guys feel just like they do. Not true. Guys have a greater sex drive and respond to visual stimulants far more than females. I'm not saying females aren't visually stimulated. Guys are just typically far more visual than girls. That's why most guys turn into mush if they see a woman in a small bikini. Try the same thing with a man in a Speedo . . . women will laugh more than lust. But guys really struggle with lust. That's why females really need to . . .

2. Discover How to Dress Modestly

When girls wear revealing clothes . . . it drives guys crazy! Just because a guy is noticing you doesn't mean he likes you. If only we could put hidden microphones in guys' locker rooms and let girls hear the way guys talk about them. Soon females would know that they are merely objects to many of these guys. Don't let any guy lower you to this level. You are so much more than just a sex object. Your value goes way beyond dressing sexy. That's why you need to . . .

3. Learn to Beware

Sadly, most girls don't realize how dangerous it is to get alone with guys. Don't go to a guy's house when his parents are gone, even if it's "just to do homework." Even if you think you don't need to flee these kinds of situations, trust me, guys do. So help them flee by not getting alone with them. In the same way, guys can't give girls a backrub without secretly wishing they could be touching much more than your back! Girls might think this sounds ridiculous. Why? They don't understand the mind of a guy (please reread point number one above). So help guys flee these situations and don't get alone with them.

4. Find a Mentor You Can Talk With About Sex

Don't travel this journey alone. Find a trustworthy adult female who will be an encouragement to you in your decision to stay sexually pure. Share your temptations and struggles. And if a guy is pushing you to do something you don't want to do, share it with this adult.

5. Run Toward Good Relationships

When the Bible tells us to flee something, it often also informs us what we can pursue instead. Hebrews 12:1–2 tells us to let go of "the sin that so easily entangles" us and "fix our eyes on Jesus" (NIV 1984). So if you need to flee a bad relationship, seek out healthy male relationships instead. Spend time with your dad or your grandfather, someone who treats you with selfless love and respect. Seek out good male friendships with Christian guys who encourage you in your faith and see you as more than just a sex object.

6. Avoid Alcohol

I can't possibly talk about girls fleeing without bringing up the subject of alcohol. Alcohol and dating don't mix. When girls drink, they lose their inhibitions. In other words, they have less control of their ability to make wise decisions. Thus, alcohol and fleeing *definitely* do not mix.

I just spoke at a convention with a few hundred military and prison chaplains in attendance. In my presentation about youth culture, attitudes, and trends, I spent some time talking about teen drinking. It's no surprise so many teens drink: We glorify it in most of our entertainment but rarely talk about consequences.

After my presentation a military chaplain told me that he and his team looked back over all their sexual assault cases over the last decade and discovered that every single one of them included alcohol. Truly 100 percent. No exception.

This isn't an anomaly. The Center of Alcohol Studies at Rutgers University tackled a research project (posted in *The Journal of Studies on Alcohol and Drugs*) following hundreds of young women from their senior year in high school through their freshman year of college. The study made two alarming discoveries:

- "Of women who had never drunk heavily in high school (if at all), nearly half admitted to binge drinking at least once by the end of their first college semester."

- "Of all young women whose biggest binge had included four to six drinks, one quarter said they'd been sexually victimized in the fall semester. That included anything from unwanted sexual contact to rape. And the more alcohol those binges involved, the greater the likelihood of sexual assault. Of women who'd ever consumed 10 or more drinks in a sitting since starting college, 59% were sexually victimized by the end of their first semester."[4]

These results are frightening on two levels. First, it's alarming to discover that almost half of female college freshmen exercised their newfound freedom by engaging in a very risky behavior. Binge drinking is no joke. It's not just having a beer or a glass of wine. Binge drinking is drinking to get drunk. This isn't surprising, considering the media messages we see and hear every day. Think about it. We are bombarded with the "drink it up" and "raise your glass" messages from almost every entertainment media source. But how many consequences do these sources show? When is the last time you saw the star of your latest sitcom get raped or sexually victimized?

The consequences many of these girls endured is even more terrifying. Rape or sexual victimization is a nightmare and often life changing. And to think that anywhere from 25 to 59 percent of these women experienced this as a result of their binge is sobering. Literally.

How can we expect to flee when we're drunk or passed out?

But these kinds of tragedies don't only occur when alcohol is involved. Sometimes girls put themselves in danger even when they have all their inhibitions. In my twenty-plus years of working with teenagers I've seen countless girls get alone with guys, completely unaware that this guy wasn't going to take no for an answer.

Girls, don't get alone with any guy. The guy could be a great guy who is just struggling with sexual temptation, or he could be a predator. Don't get alone with either.

After two decades of studying youth culture and hanging out with teenagers, here's what I've observed about young girls today:

They know enough about being sexy to attract guys . . . but not enough to beware.

Are you "fleeing" sexual situations?

Ask yourself what kind of guy you want. Do you want a guy who just wants to use you sexually? Or do you want a guy who values you as a whole person? It's this simple: If guys care about you for more than just sex, then they won't mind hanging out with you in public.

A Word for the Guys—What Fleeing Looks Like (Girls, You Can Spy in on This Too)

Sexual temptation is a huge lure for young men. Whether it's porn, masturbation, hooking up for casual sex, or the pressure they feel when they get alone with their girlfriends, today's young men feel enticed by sexual temptation recurrently.

It's no surprise with the abundance of sexually charged images and messages bombarding us daily, if not hourly. Most young people are inundated with stimuli encouraging them to think sexual thoughts and act out in some way.

In the next chapter I'll talk specifically about pornography and masturbation, and how to flee those temptations. So for this few pages, let's focus mostly on fleeing sexual temptation with your girlfriend, and/or the girls you encounter day to day.

The Bible tells us to flee "youthful lusts" (2 Timothy 2:22) and specifically "sexual immorality" (1 Corinthians 6:18). What does this look like each day for guys?

1. Look Ahead

It happens like this: A pretty girl walks by. What do most guys do? They turn their heads and take a closer look (and they usually aren't checking out her hairstyle). I told my son, "Don't feel guilty if you notice a pretty girl . . . but leave it at that. When you turn for that second look, it's usually lusting." He didn't argue, because he knows it's true.

2. Browse Publicly

Doctors recommend parents shouldn't allow computers or smartphones in their kids' bedrooms. Instead, they say put a computer out in a family area and monitor their kids' computer use. Why would doctors recommend this? Probably because they know the temptations that private late-night browsing can cause. Don't put yourself in tempting situations. Browsing an unmonitored computer with no adults around is a good way to open yourself up to temptation and one of the reasons that porn is such a problem for guys in this country.

3. Don't Get Alone With a Girl

Every bit of entertainment we watch seems to sell us on the fact that guys should always invite a girl up or park with her or seek other scenarios where they can be alone. If you follow most of these situations to their natural conclusion, sex is the result. Getting alone with a girl is flirting with disaster.

4. Talk About It

I recommended this to girls, and I emphasize it even more so for guys. Don't travel this journey alone. Find a trustworthy adult male who will be an encouragement to you in your decision to stay sexually pure. Find someone you can be honest with and share your temptations and struggles. The Bible encourages us to "confess [our] sins to each other" so we can be healed (James 5:16). We guys need mentors and friends who can hold us accountable.

Run Away

Paul warns us about a lot of sins in the New Testament: gossip, anger, bitterness, stealing, drunkenness, even acting generally foolish. But rarely does he literally instruct us to "run away" or "flee" from these sins as he does lust and sexual temptation.

Do you think we should listen?

If we're told that we shouldn't put our toothbrush within six feet of the toilet because of airborne particles . . . most of us will probably store our toothbrush about twenty feet away if possible. Why? Because the thought of poop fumes or pee splashes wandering onto our toothbrush is *not acceptable*!

There is a principle here: If we discover danger to be within a certain proximity, we avoid that proximity completely.

Why don't we do that with sexual temptation? We determine we don't even want to start the process . . . then we go and put ourselves in situations where the process not only starts, but it's hard to stop!

Why flirt with disaster?

No, I'm not saying that you shouldn't hold hands with your boyfriend or girlfriend. I'm not even saying you shouldn't kiss him or her. I'm simply drawing attention to the overt truth of the Bible, which lays out God's design clearly.

Be careful not to initiate the launch sequence. Save the amazing process of sex for your spouse when you get married. Flee sexual temptation.

And today, one of the biggest sexual temptations is pornography, so let's take a closer look at the lure of porn in the next chapter.

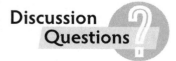

Discussion Questions

1. This chapter shared some pretty sobering studies about the effects of music and entertainment media. Why do

you think teens who listen to raunchy sexual lyrics start having sex sooner?

2. Why do you think teens who viewed movies with sexual content were profoundly influenced by what they watched, so much so that they initiated sexual behavior earlier than their peers who had viewed less sexual content, and even tended to imitate the on-screen sexual behaviors they saw?

3. Then why do young people often say, "This music/TV show/movie doesn't affect me?"

4. We read several ways guys and girls can flee sexual temptation and lust. Which piece of advice for girls did you think was the most relevant? Explain.

5. What impacted you the most about the Center of Alcohol Studies research project concerning girls' binge drinking when they get to college?

6. What are some of the consequences this study uncovered?

7. Why are heavy drinkers more likely to experience sexual assault or unwanted sexual contact? How does alcohol affect your ability to flee?

8. Do you think most of these young women foresaw these consequences? Why or why not?

9. Which piece of advice for guys did you think was the most relevant? Explain.

10. Why is getting alone with a girl "flirting with disaster"?

11. What is one action that would help you flee sexual temptation?

12. Who is someone you can talk with more to help you with this?

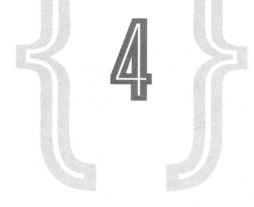

The Lure of Porn
and Masturbation

t's hilarious. Just search for it on Google Images."

That's how it started.

"Chris" was only twelve years old when his friend told him about the funny meme. But what started as an innocent search quickly led down a rabbit trail to hard-core porn.

Chris had actually never stumbled on any pornographic images before, probably because his parents had tried to be really careful. They didn't have porn filters on the family computer, but it rested on a desk in the great room adjoining the TV and the kitchen, and Mom or Dad were always right there when Chris browsed the web.

But this particular afternoon Chris's dad was still at work and his mom was running errands. Chris didn't think anything about booting up the computer alone in the house. He had done it before. And today he was simply curious about the funny picture his friend had described.

A quick click of the mouse, a few taps of his fingers on the keyboard, and he was browsing through Google Images looking for the funny meme. In the third row of pictures, second from the right, a picture of a girl wearing a bikini appeared. The caption was enticing.

Chris's heart rate accelerated, and he shifted in the squeaky computer chair. He looked over his shoulder. No one was there. He knew that but couldn't help but double check.

He slowly scrolled the cursor over to the right, landing on the picture of the girl. A quick click and he was looking at the image full size. A button invited him to visit the page the picture originated from.

He stared at the picture for a moment, taking it all in. He had seen pictures of girls in bikinis before, but they had only really started to interest him in the last year. Plus, this girl was truly mesmerizing. Her bikini top barely covered all she had—and she had plenty. Her smile was enticing, especially the way she was licking her lips ever so slightly.

Chris didn't wait another second. He clicked on Visit Page.

One click led to another, and less than five minutes later Chris was watching a video of two girls doing things he had never even dreamed about. It was his first exposure to hardcore pornography, actually his first time exposed to porn of any kind. But sadly, it wasn't his last. Within a few months Chris was seeking out porn daily, unable to break free from the grip it had on him.

Chris isn't alone. We live in a world where porn is seeping through every digital and analog signal crawling through our homes. Sometimes it's difficult to dodge many of the temptations we see every day.

First Exposure

I'll never forget my first exposure to a pornographic video. This was a long time ago in a world without the Internet or Blu-ray players, but sexual temptation was available regardless. I was at my friend's house and he pulled a VHS tape off the shelf with the label *The Battle of Britain*. With a smirk on his face he asked, "Do you want to see something?" I had a good feeling we weren't going to watch *The Battle of Britain*.

He opened his top-loading VCR, a relatively new gadget at the time, inserted *The Battle of Britain*, and hit Fast-Forward. He watched the counter and eventually hit Play.

In the moments to follow I watched my first porno.

I was thirteen years old.

It was much like one of those soft-core porn movies they show on late-night Cinemax or Showtime today. Completely naked people having sex. Everything but extreme close-ups.

Those came a year later.

Age fourteen. Same friend, same house, same VCR, no parents, just my friend and me. He pulled the World War II film *Tora! Tora! Tora!* off of his shelf.

He smirked. "Do you want to see something?"

Yeah, it wasn't *Tora! Tora! Tora!*

Moments later we were watching hard-core porn. This was thirty years ago, and I can still remember explicit details of this film. I remember the title, and I remember the name of the female porn star. I got to know her well in the next few months, because every chance I had I was over at my friend's house watching the tape labeled *Tora! Tora! Tora!* over and over again.

I learned a lot about human anatomy from that ninety-minute film, and even more about the lure of sexual temptation.

As I reflect back on this experience, I remember being magnetically drawn to the visuals of this film. I couldn't get enough of it. It was the most arousing feeling I had ever experienced. That's probably why I always disappeared to the bathroom immediately after the film to do what most young boys do when they crave sexual release.

Then the guilt would kick in.

But a day later, a week later . . . whenever I could get over to my friend's house . . . I did it again. It was a cycle. *Tora! Tora! Tora!* . . . masturbate . . . feel guilty . . . *Tora! Tora! Tora!* . . . masturbate . . . feel guilty. . . .

Then one day my friend's dad randomly decided he wanted to watch a war movie, *Tora! Tora! Tora!* . . . and that was the end of that.

Today Porn Is Everywhere

In my world, it wasn't easy to find porn. I had to search for it, and then sneak behind the backs of adults to watch it. With the exception of my *Tora! Tora! Tora!* binge, it probably only happened a couple times a year. If I had been offered an avenue to see more, I'm embarrassed to admit, I might have traveled that road every day, perhaps multiple times.

Today porn bombards us through every cable and signal permeating our homes. Unless we all shut off the power grid and move to a shack in the mountains, porn is readily accessible.

If you have the Internet, the most depraved forms of porn are just a click away. If you ever stay in a hotel with your family, you probably have noticed hard-core porn is always one of the TV's main menu choices. If your family is one of the 91 percent of Americans who pay for TV reception at home, soft-core porn is available on far too many channels.

Maybe that's why so many teenagers have looked at porn:

- 93 percent of boys and 62 percent of girls are exposed to porn before their eighteenth birthday.[1]
- 71 percent of teenagers feel the need to hide their online activity from parents.[2]
- 15 percent of boys and 9 percent of girls have viewed (illegal) child pornography online.[3]

If you are eleven or older, chances are you have already stumbled upon it at least once.

So how can we flee the grip of porn?

Fleeing Porn

Maybe you've only stumbled on porn once or twice, or perhaps it's been far more than that. Maybe you haven't even encountered it at all, but you know it's out there. Regardless, porn is a very common temptation that beckons many of us like a big bag of Halloween candy. How can we possibly resist this temptation?

Let's look at three effective ways we can find deliverance from porn.

1. Understand the Truth About Sex

We've been talking about God's gift of sex throughout this whole book, but specifically in chapter 1, "Why Wait?" Remember, sex is an amazing gift you can share with your spouse someday, and that's a gift worth waiting for.

Allow me to address the guys for a moment. Guys, if you're tempted to look at a naked woman it's understandable. The reason you want to look at a naked woman is because God created you to enjoy looking at a naked woman . . . *one* naked woman.

Don't get me wrong, guys. I'm not saying it's okay to look at a bunch of naked women. I'm actually telling you just the opposite. God created you so that someday when you find the right woman and commit to her in marriage, you'll get enjoyment just looking at *her*! It's been that way since the very beginning.

Remember in Genesis 2:18 when God said, "It is not good for the man to be alone"? While Adam was sleeping, God made him a wife. Adam woke up, saw this beautiful naked woman, and said, "At last!" (v. 23).

So the two of them got to hang out together in the garden . . . *naked*. And it was good: "Now the man and his wife were both naked, but they felt no shame" (Genesis 2:25).

Sadly, sin crept into the world, and when that happened people started trying to pervert God's creation. They took something that was good and they twisted it from its design. A husband and wife were supposed to enjoy each other naked, but when sin entered the world, man started thinking, "Hey . . . if my wife looks good naked, I bet I could experience even more fun by being with other naked women also."

The Bible warns us of this, reminding us of God's original plan between husband and wife. Remember what we read in Proverbs 5:

> Let your wife be a fountain of blessing for you.
> Rejoice in the wife of your youth.
> She is a loving deer, a graceful doe.
> Let her breasts satisfy you always.
> May you always be captivated by her love.
>
> vv. 18–19

Let me ask you:

- Who does God say is a blessing for us?
- What should we let satisfy us always?

Let's keep reading:

> Why be captivated, my son, by an immoral woman,
> or fondle the breasts of a promiscuous woman?
> For the Lord sees clearly what a man does,
> examining every path he takes.
> An evil man is held captive by his own sins;
> they are ropes that catch and hold him.
> He will die for lack of self-control;
> he will be lost because of his great foolishness.
>
> vv. 20–23

Let me ask you:

- Who should we not be captivated by or attracted to?
- Whose breasts aren't for us?
- Where are some places we might encounter these kinds of distractions today, the breasts of women who aren't our wives?
- What are some of the "ropes that catch and hold" us?
- What will happen to us if we lack self-control?

God wants us to enjoy sex with our spouse someday, and that gift of sex was created to be shared between one man and one woman. Just like sleeping with someone before you're married lingers into marriage, porn brings others into the marriage bed. Porn creates unreal expectations. Porn becomes a rope or snare that catches us and holds us captive from the freedom God provides in our lives.

Plus, let's be honest. Porn leads to lust, and we know lust is wrong (we'll examine those passages again a little closer in a few pages when we talk about masturbation).

The truth is God wants us to enjoy looking at one person naked, our spouse. When we go outside of that design, consequences occur.

And that brings us to the second way we can find deliverance from the grip of porn . . .

2. Recognize Natural Consequences

When people are engaging in temporary pleasures, they don't often pay attention to long-term consequences. In other words, when someone is enjoying pornographic pictures, they aren't typically thinking about why they might regret this activity the following day, the following week, or the following year. But consequences have a way of creeping up on us.

I knew a teenager named Nick. When Nick first started looking at pornographic pictures he didn't think it would harm anyone, but his occasional browsing turned into an addiction he couldn't quit, affecting his family, his girlfriend, and his relationship with God. After years of trying to quit, he eventually got married, thinking the problem would go away. Several years after he was married he got caught browsing porn at his workplace. His wife was devastated and he eventually had to go to counseling to escape his addiction.

But that's the way many of us respond to temptations. We think, "It won't happen to me." We don't look realistically at the consequences . . . like impotence. This isn't a scare tactic, this is just the truth. The fact is, impotence is increasing, and many men are not satisfied with their sexual partner (I'd love to say "wife" here, but unfortunately, for many it's just "sexual partner") because they're truly becoming addicted to the never-ending stream of dopamine spikes they get from watching different girls do different things at the click of a button.[4]

The more porn guys watch, the more difficult it is to become turned on. This is becoming a huge problem with young men, *Psychology Today* explains,

Desperate young men from various cultures, with different levels of education, religiosity, attitudes, values, diets, marijuana use, and personalities are seeking help. They have only two things in common: heavy use of today's Internet porn and increasing need for more extreme material.[5]

This is much different than the *Playboy* magazines men looked at just a decade ago. The static images of *Playboy* can't compete with the readily available high-speed connection to the biggest database of porn in the world—the world wide web. Men are literally "numbing their brain's normal response to pleasure," and they can't "get it up" for their sexual partner anymore.[6]

I don't know about you, but I find that scary! I don't want to fail in the bedroom because of an "affair" with virtual women on the screens in my house. Impotence is a natural consequence that I'd rather avoid. I think most teenagers would agree.

Porn has other natural consequences, like convincing girls they are sex objects. Porn sites communicate two major lies to teenage girls: You need to look perfect, and your value is based on sex. Porn is "sexualizing" you, just as we talked about in the previous chapter. Porn doesn't care if you're a good singer or a good volleyball player. . . . It only values you if you are sexy.

Girls, you are so much more than a sex object. Watch out for porn. It will convince you otherwise.

Real love takes work, patience, self-sacrifice, tenderness, and compassion. Real relationships are so much more than just sex. Porn, however, is just a sex show where perfect-looking models engage in pure animalistic thrill with no concern for the long-term. Porn sets false expectations all around and eventually leads to disappointment with reality.

Let's look at a third way we can find deliverance from porn . . .

3. Establish Safeguards and Accountability

If you have already discovered porn, ask yourself: Where and when did you look at it? What do you think would be good safeguards you or your family could put into place to help you flee this temptation? Is there a channel you need to ask your parents to block? Is there a parental control you need Mom or Dad to implement? What about when you get out of the house and live on your own? What could you do to flee sexual temptation then? Is there a TV channel you should avoid subscribing to?

Paul repeatedly instructed us to flee sexual sin. What does that look like in your world?

Porn is a powerful enemy that seeks to destroy anyone it can get in its clutches, and porn often leads to masturbation. Let's talk briefly about masturbation.

What About Masturbation?

Masturbation is sexual self-gratification. In other words, it is touching your own genitals for sexual pleasure.

Masturbation is a huge struggle for young people today. A recent study by the National Survey of Sexual Health and Behavior (NSSHB) reported:

- "For both sexes, the likelihood of engaging in masturbation appeared to increase with age."

- "Among boys between the ages of 14 and 17 the percentage of those who had masturbated at least once rose from about 63 to 80 percent."

- "Among girls, those figures were lower but still followed an upward slope, rising from about 43 percent to 58 percent across the same time-frame."[7]

Let me just say, I've met very few men (just a couple, actually) who told me they *didn't* masturbate regularly in their teen years. The percentages are very high for boys. I think they are easily in the 80 to 90 percentile.

This isn't surprising. Males are more visual than females in a world overflowing with sexually charged images, and the male sex drive is strong . . . out of control, at times.

This doesn't mean females have no sex drive. Some are very driven by sex, and others experiment, curious about something so desired by most of the world.

Regardless of the exact numbers, it seems that over half of young people, both male and female, are doing it.

Plus, today's young people are waiting until their late 20s, on average, to get married and must resist sexual temptation far longer. Fewer of today's twentysomethings are married than any generation prior at the same age. A 2014 PewResearch report revealed that only a quarter of Millennials (26 percent) are married. When previous generations were the age that Millennials are now, 36 percent of Generation X, 48 percent of Baby Boomers and 65 percent of the members of the Silent Generation were married.[8]

Grandma and Grandpa didn't have to wait as long for sex. And they didn't have to dodge porn on every screen either.

Let's just say masturbation seems like a solution for many. Not to mention that our world doesn't see any problem with it.

Is the world right?

Is masturbation a big deal?

Innocent Exploration?

Once kids hit puberty, some might discover that it feels good when they touch their genitals and they might experiment with it. This could start out as a pretty innocent act. Many young people would describe it by saying, "It tickles."

Again, this often can be an innocent exploration of the human body, and it contrasts greatly with the person who is viewing porn, lusting, and masturbating.

I remember the first time I discovered something "tingly" below the waist. I was about eleven years old. I hadn't gone through puberty (I was a late bloomer—all of my friends had body hair before I did), but I realized it felt good when I rubbed my penis a certain way in the sheets of my bed. Sometimes I found myself doing it until I reached orgasm.

I didn't do this every day and I really don't recall thinking about girls or the female body when I did it. I just remember it feeling good.

By sixth grade my interest in the fairer sex had increased significantly. Sexual imagery began catching my eye, and I was distracted when my female classmates wore tight or revealing clothing.

I can't tell you the exact moment, but masturbation quickly became a sexual thing for me. It wasn't just some innocent tingly feeling anymore. I thought about girls when I masturbated, and by thirteen, as I shared earlier in the chapter, I was viewing or thinking about pornographic images and those eventually led me to masturbate.

The mind is a powerful thing.

At this point, the act of masturbation always made me feel guilty. I knew what lust was . . . *and I was definitely lusting.*

It became a habit, something I continued through most of my teen years. It's something I never brought up to anyone, something I was embarrassed by, but it was also something I really wanted deliverance from.

Looking for Answers

My dad subscribed me to a Christian magazine at the time, *Campus Life*. Each issue had a column about sex. Every time I received an issue I immediately turned to the sex column and read what the author had to say. He occasionally addressed issues like lust, but rarely mentioned masturbation. I was always disappointed with what I read because the author never addressed the specific questions I had.

No one used the words I had heard.

No one addressed the thoughts I had had.

No one was willing to talk about the truth in explicit detail.

My guess is that you or your friends have numerous unanswered questions about this topic. I know, because every time I talk to young people about the subject, they always approach me and ask me questions at the end of my talk. And whenever I offer a question box where young people can ask anonymous questions, they always ask about masturbation.

I find that today's young believers have two major questions about masturbation:

1. Is masturbation wrong?

2. If it is wrong, how can I stop?

Let's look at these answers explicitly.

Is Masturbation Wrong?

The Bible doesn't address masturbation specifically, but it clearly addresses lust.

We've talked about God's way in previous chapters, so no need to rehash everything. But let's look at the highlights and then specifically at lust.

As we know, God's plan was made clear in the garden: a husband and a wife are to be united as one in the flesh. But some people didn't want to stick to their own spouses. They wanted others too, or they didn't want to wait for marriage. So

God made it obvious, starting with the Ten Commandments in Exodus 20:14: "You must not commit adultery."

That's pretty clear. Don't have sex outside of marriage.

Then in the New Testament, the apostle Paul communicates on the topic clearly in many passages, very explicitly in 1 Corinthians 6:18: "Run from sexual sin! No other sin so clearly affects the body as this one does. For sexual immorality is a sin against your own body."

Again, the term *sexual sin* means "the voluntary sex of an unmarried person." In other words, run from any temptation to have sex with someone if you're not married to them. Paul uses this term multiple times throughout his letters in the New Testament, usually saying something like flee from it, or have nothing to do with it.

But sadly, humans always try to come up with excuses for our sins. That's what the religious people did back in Jesus' day. They thought they could get away with just *thinking* about sex, as long as they didn't actually do it. Jesus himself decided to address this, calling it lust, and labeling it just as bad as adultery.

> You have heard the commandment that says, "You must not commit adultery." But I say, anyone who even looks at a woman with lust has already committed adultery with her in his heart. So if your eye—even your good eye—causes you to lust, gouge it out and throw it away. It is better for you to lose one part of your body than for your whole body to be thrown into hell.
>
> Matthew 5:27–29

Jesus wasn't known for tiptoeing around issues. He was loving, he was merciful, he was forgiving . . . but when it came to religious people trying to justify their sins, he was forthright and frank. *Don't lust. You might as well have sex with someone who is not your wife, because it's the exact same thing. I look at the heart, not the fake actions you parade around!*

Paul chimes in on the same idea, advising us to flee any "youthful lusts":

Run from anything that stimulates youthful lusts. Instead, pursue righteous living, faithfulness, love, and peace. Enjoy the companionship of those who call on the Lord with pure hearts.

2 Timothy 2:22

So we know that sex was created for marriage, sex outside of marriage is wrong, and if we think we are being good because we just imagine having sex with someone we aren't married to . . . *we should pluck our eyes out*!

So let me ask you. Is masturbating while looking at porn wrong?

The answer is pretty clear. Lusting is wrong. If we think we're not sinning when we look at or imagine pictures of people we're not married to, then we're fooling ourselves.

Let me say it again. Lusting is wrong. If we lust while masturbating, then it's wrong.

Now, I've met the occasional person who tells me, "I don't lust when I masturbate. It just feels good."

Here's my opinion about that:

If you're a guy, you're not only an adulterer, you're now also a liar. The male plumbing doesn't work that way. We don't achieve orgasm while thinking about Hannibal marching across the Alps with his elephants. I've talked with countless teenagers about masturbation in my twenty-plus years of youth ministry, listening to their candid confessions, and have never encountered a kid who thought about his geometry homework while masturbating. He might have been thinking about curves . . . *but not the ones in geometry class.*

Guys lust when they masturbate. End of story.

Sure, if a married guy masturbates while thinking of his wife, then that's not sin. God knows our hearts and our minds. He knows exactly what we're thinking about. If we're lusting about someone other than our wife . . . it's sin.

I've also heard single guys argue, "I'm thinking about my future wife when I masturbate, so it's okay."

Again, I realize that this is a difficult temptation. But let's not distort truth to rationalize our sin.

The fact is, if you're thinking about someone who is your "future wife" . . . she ain't your wife yet. If a cop caught you looking in her window, you couldn't argue, "But that's my wife!"

The officer of the law would ask you, "Then why are you out here in the bushes looking in her window if that's your wife?"

"Well . . . it's my future wife."

Try that one sometime with a cop and see how far it gets you. (And God's a little smarter than most cops . . . no disrespect to my friends in blue.)

As for girls, I'll be bold enough to say that lust is usually the primary factor. Can I say without a doubt that is always the case? I'm a male, so I'll have to say the jury is still out on this one. Many females admit to thinking about erotic situations while they masturbate, but many also claim to be "just spacing out."

The female body works much differently than the male. Males strive for a climax, and once they orgasm, they're done. Guys are all about the climax. Females can be more sensitive throughout the whole act. They might climax multiple times, or sadly, not at all. Some females claim that masturbating with a shower nozzle just feels good, massages, or tickles.

Some females argue that women who masturbate are just filling a void or have attachment issues. Others in the Christian community have spoken out against these claims, like Jordan Monge in her *Christianity Today* article, "The Real Problem with Female Masturbation." The subtitle of the article is "Call it what it is: Ladies who lust."

Monge contends,

> We need a strategy that recognizes the sin of lust and calls it by its name, rather than pretending that women have no agency beyond reacting to environmental stressors or psychological difficulties. We must treat lust like other sins—not a way we act out as a consequence of other problems in our lives—but as a sin requiring us to learn the discipline of self-control that we must master if we ever hope to be the women God made us to be.[9]

I'm not going to point any fingers, because I can't tell a female how she feels. But I can say this: If we are lusting, we need to call it what it is. More important, we need to look for ways to flee these temptations.

Breaking Free

So how can you break free from the temptation to masturbate?

Let me ask a bigger question: Who's driving?

If your heart had a driver's seat and a steering wheel . . . who would be in that driver's seat?

Many of us put our own selfish desires in that driver's seat. We drive where we want, doing what we want at any given moment. Sadly, we are being chauffeured around by our sinful nature. When we let our sinful nature drive, our lives often reflect it. We don't flee sexual sin; we welcome it. I have a feeling if most of us looked at our phones it would be quite evident. Our playlists are full of sexually charged lyrics, and the images on our screens are full of racy visuals and "do what feels right at the moment" messages.

What do you think "feels right" when we encounter sexual temptations in the moment?

The key to fighting sexual sin is to let God drive. We can't do it on our own; we need the power God gives us through a relationship with him and his Spirit living inside of us. The world loves to tell us to do whatever *we desire*. God's Word tells us to *let his Spirit guide us*.

> So I say, let the Holy Spirit guide your lives. Then you won't be doing what your sinful nature craves. The sinful nature wants to do evil, which is just the opposite of what the Spirit wants. And the Spirit gives us desires that are the opposite of what the sinful nature desires.
>
> Galatians 5:16–17

Are we listening to God, or our own desires?

John Piper provides some pretty good advice about battling lust in a very memorable acronym, ANTHEM.[10] His suggestions include avoiding temptation, saying no to lustful thoughts, and turning our minds toward Christ. Google "John Piper, ANTHEM" for the full explanation.

Are you avoiding tempting situations?

Who are you letting drive?

Discussion Questions

1. What was Adam's reaction when he saw Eve naked? Why do you think God made us this way?

2. In this chapter we looked at a passage of Scripture in Proverbs 5 and asked several questions about those verses. Answer each of those questions now.

3. Those verses talked about being "held captive" by our own sin, particularly sexual temptations. What is one of the biggest sexual temptations that seems to "hold" or trap guys today?

4. How can girls be "held captive" by these temptations too?

5. What are some of the natural consequences guys can experience when they regularly look at porn?

6. What do girls commonly learn from pornography? In other words, what does porn communicate to girls?

7. Is masturbation wrong? Explain.

8. Read the following passage of Scripture:

Run from anything that stimulates youthful lusts. Instead, pursue righteous living, faithfulness, love, and peace. Enjoy the companionship of those who call on the Lord with pure hearts.

2 Timothy 2:22

What does this passage tell us to run from? What are some modern-day examples of "anything that stimulates youthful lusts"?

9. What does the verse say we should pursue instead? How can we pursue these things? Give an example.

10. What are some tempting situations God might want you to avoid?

11. How can you let God help you do this?

12. Is there someone you can talk with who can help you with this?

5

Tough Questions

s it okay if I masturbate to keep from looking at porn?"
    "Is it wrong if I am attracted to someone of the same
    sex?"
    "I just want to be loved, and the only way guys want me
is if I give them sex. Does God want me to be alone?"

These are the kinds of questions asked by many young people
today . . . and these questions, and more, are exactly what we're
going to answer in this chapter.

Is it okay to send each other sexy pictures on our phones?

My guess is you already know the answer to this question.

Sure, the Bible *doesn't* say, "Thou shalt not sendeth naked
pictures." True. But let's break this down from what we know
the Bible *does* say.

If a girl sends her boyfriend a sexy picture, he is going to be tempted to lust, and lust is sin. We are supposed to flee this kind of temptation.

If a guy is sending a girl a sexy picture, first, he's confused. Most girls aren't visual like this. But second, if a girl is actually turned on by this, then she's lusting, and then she shouldn't be doing it.

Sadly, a recent study showed that over half of teenagers have received or sent either sexually suggestive texts ("I think your body is hot") or pictures.[1] Similar studies show those teens are four to six times more likely to have sex than those teens who don't.[2] Think about it. If you're thinking about sex and flirting with your girlfriend or boyfriend with sexually explicit messages, those actions eventually progress to something more—the complete opposite of fleeing sexual temptation.

So no, don't send sexy pictures until you're married. And even then, be careful sending sexy pictures to your spouse, because you don't ever want those pictures getting out. Save that kind of fun for the bedroom, where there's no chance of pictures showing up on the Internet someday and ruining your life.

Can I have sex when I'm engaged, or when I'm really sure I'm going to be with this person forever?

This is another great question, and it's usually asked by someone who doesn't necessarily want to know the truth as much as they want to find some justification for their actions. How do I know this? Because not only have I addressed this question from young people countless times . . . *I asked this question myself when I was engaged!* (And I only wanted to hear one answer.)

Sometimes young people will even arm themselves with verses to support their claim. And in today's world, they can Google it and find someone who argues premarital sex for engaged couples. Their logic usually sounds something like this:

> In Bible times the betrothal period was very much like our engagement, and as we know from Deuteronomy 20:7, it's okay to sleep with our fiancé during this period. We've both been pure so far, so now that we've found that special someone and have committed to each other in this engagement, isn't it okay to go ahead and share that intimate bond? After all, it's for two people who want to spend the rest of their lives together, right? And we are exactly that! Who says we need to wait for a piece of paper when it's really God who joins us together?

Yeah . . . I've heard all of that, including the bad interpretation of the Deuteronomy verse.

First, let's be clear. God's plan for marriage is unmistakable in the Bible. Reread chapter 1 of this book. It's all laid out. Husband and wife. Not fiancés. Not people who really love each other and have "promised" each other.

Second, the betrothal period was way more serious than an engagement. It's hardly a comparison. It was a very serious commitment, so much so that you actually had to divorce to get out of it. You might recall the example of Mary and Joseph. Joseph was "pledged to be married" to Mary (Matthew 1:18 NIV), but then she got pregnant. "Because Joseph her husband was faithful to the law, and yet did not want to expose her to public disgrace, he had in mind to divorce her quietly" (Matthew 1:19 NIV).

This "divorce" was from the betrothal. Serious stuff.

Third, it wasn't God's plan for betrothed couples to have sex. People might try to cite verses like Deuteronomy 20:7 that seem like exceptions. But look up that verse for yourself. Depending on the version you have, it will read something like this:

Has anyone here just become engaged to a woman but not yet married her? Well, you may go home and get married! You might die in the battle, and someone else would marry her.

Deuteronomy 20:7

Some think that this can be interpreted as "go home and sleep with her."

It's funny how people love to try to find one exception from an Old Testament civil or ceremonial law and use it as the justification for their actions rather than seeking what God's Word says repeatedly throughout Scripture: *No sex outside of marriage, either adultery or sexual immorality.* In chapter 1 of this book we looked at numerous verses sharing this truth, including Hebrews 13:4, addressing both adultery and fornication: "Marriage should be honored by all, and the marriage bed kept pure, for God will judge the adulterer and all the sexually immoral" (Hebrews 13:4 NIV).

Fourth (yeah, I even have a fourth reason), I've met countless couples who were engaged only to break up before the wedding. This just happened to a close friend of ours. What then?

Sex is reserved for marriage. Not engagement, not some exception of betrothal . . . *just marriage.*

So if you want to have sex with your fiancé, then get married.

Is it wrong to lie in a bed, but not have sex, with your significant other?

Let's be honest. Men have a huge sex drive, and I don't know a single man who wouldn't be tempted lying in bed with a female.

The Bible repeatedly says, "Flee sexual immorality." Lying in a bed together is the complete opposite of fleeing. This would tempt any man with a pulse.

If marriage is for one man and one woman, how come so many Bible heroes had multiple wives?

God's plan was laid out clearly in the garden. One man, one woman, to become one in the flesh. That plan never changed. But people strayed from God's plan regardless.

The Old Testament stories often tell us all the explicit details, but within those details lies the truth.

For example: Abraham didn't trust God's promise for a son, so he slept with Hagar. Seem like no big deal? This single decision caused fighting, jealousy, and chaos that has lasted for thousands of years.

Jacob was tricked into his first marriage, so he married again. When those two wives didn't produce like Jacob wanted, he slept with two other women. These decisions caused competition, quarreling, and jealousy for generations to come.

God instructed his kings to be an example to God's people and only take one wife (Deuteronomy 17:14–20). Most of them didn't, and the result was consequences of the worst kind.

God's plan for one husband and one wife is clearly the best plan.

Whenever someone really investigates the Scripture, it's plainly evident that God's way is so much better than our way. The Old Testament stories demonstrate that.

At the same time, these stories demonstrate that God can use sinful people, blemishes and all. Yes, these people would have avoided many natural consequences had they listened to God in the first place. But God uses us despite our mistakes.

What counts as "sex" anyway?

I will reiterate what we covered pretty clearly in chapter 2 of this book. Sex isn't just intercourse, it's an intimate process that begins when people "activate the launch sequence." Anyone who has ever been in a moment of passion, even with all their clothes on, would attest to the intensity and heat of the moment. It's difficult to stop, simply because it's a process that's not supposed to be stopped. Anyone in that situation is clearly thinking sexual thoughts, and those moments are supposed to be reserved for marriage. When sexual thoughts are outside of marriage, they are lust.

So call me crazy when I label it *sexual immorality* when two teenagers lie down on a couch with their clothes on and make out passionately. Some thought Jesus was crazy when he told them, "But I say, anyone who even looks at a woman with lust has already committed adultery with her in his heart" (Matthew 5:28).

So what counts as sex? Any intimate physical activity that starts the engines roaring. These moments are meant for marriage, and they're amazing!

Why would God, who says that all he created was good, tell us that we can't have sex whenever we want?

This is a great question, and it's really a matter of perspective.

You are living in a small time period of your life where sexual temptation is very difficult and very real. For my great grandpa, this was only a few years. Kids were beginning puberty later, and they were getting married earlier. He was married at eighteen. He probably only endured a few years of sexual temptation.

I began puberty a little earlier and got married at twenty. So I was tempted sexually for almost eight years.

My son went through puberty earlier than I did; he's now twenty-one and he's not close to getting married. These years might seem long and arduous for you. They might seem like torture. Why would God make you endure such suffering?

A few thoughts:

1. Don't Wait So Long for Marriage

In 1 Corinthians 7:9 Paul writes, "But if they cannot control themselves, they should marry, for it is better to marry than to burn with passion" (NIV). Today's young people seem to want to finish college and grad school and pay off loans before getting married. And one reason they aren't in a hurry to marry is because they're sleeping around anyway. That's not God's plan. If two people really want to get married, they can make it happen. It might take sacrifice, but it's possible. I know. My wife and I were twenty and twenty-one years old when we got married.

2. Don't Date Until You're Ready

You don't need an exclusive boyfriend or girlfriend when you're twelve years old (or fifteen for that matter). I know, it's hard, because every Disney channel show you watched growing up shows sixth graders pursuing dating relationships, and your friends are all pursuing them too. Dating isn't bad, but ask yourself, "Where's the future in this?" Date when you're good and ready to find a suitable companion. Until then, enjoy plenty of friends of the opposite sex.

3. Waiting for Sex Is a Discipline and Well Worth the Price

Genesis tells us the story of a man named Jacob who was so in love with the woman he wanted to marry that he worked seven years to marry her. (Then ended up working seven more.) How hard are you willing to work for the man/woman you love? How much are you willing to endure? These years might be tough, but discipline yourself to enjoy the friendship of the opposite sex until you get married, even those whom you date. Then enjoy a lifetime of great sex. The alternative is to enjoy a promiscuous lifestyle for just a few years right now, and then suffer the consequences of that promiscuity for a lifetime. Your choice.

Is premarital oral sex wrong?

If you read chapters 1 and 2 in this book, then you know the answer to this question. What does the Bible tell us about sexual acts outside of marriage?

Earlier in this book we read several verses where we were told to flee any kind of sexual immorality. If someone were to still argue that oral sex isn't sex, I would refer to Jesus' teaching that lust is adultery. And I don't know many people who can have oral sex without having sexual thoughts or lusting.

In short, oral sex is an intimate sexual act; and intimate sexual acts are reserved for marriage.

If a guy has anal sex with a girl, are they still virgins?

Anal sex is a sexual act. If a couple engages in anal sex instead of intercourse so they can stay sexually pure, they're fooling themselves. Just like oral sex, anal sex is a type of sexual activity where you are undoubtedly having sexual thoughts. If you do this outside of marriage, it's sexual immorality, which is sin.

In addition, people who have anal sex can experience some potential unwanted effects like hemorrhoids, or even tearing. It's not a popular subject to talk about, but the fact is, God made the vagina self-lubricating and perfect for the act of making love. When couples try anal sex, they usually use a lubricant, and they have to wash really well when finished. Even then, the woman might get hemorrhoids or experience tearing. Most doctors would recommend extreme caution.

Is it okay if I masturbate to keep from looking at porn?

We already discussed masturbation in the last chapter and determined that most masturbation involves lust. And we know lust is clearly wrong.

So what this question is really asking is, "Is it okay to do one sin to keep from doing another?"

Sin has consequences, period. Think how much better it would be to seek out other ways to flee porn rather than masturbating while lusting in our minds. (Flip back to the previous chapters and look once again at some of those suggestions for fleeing pornography and other sexual temptations.)

Is it good to masturbate before a date to "flee" having sex with my girlfriend?

This is almost the same question as above, but with a little added use of Scripture. Just as Satan twisted Scripture to tempt Jesus, sometimes people will twist Scripture to try to justify sins.

No, same as above. Avoiding one sin doesn't justify another. If you want to "flee" having sex with your girlfriend, avoid tempting situations. Go to dinner and then hang out with some friends. Don't get alone with her.

I just want to be loved, and the only way guys want me is if I give them sex. Does God want me to be alone?

In chapter 2, I made a statement:

Guys give love to get sex.
Girls give sex to get love.

No, not all guys are evil manipulators, and no, not all girls are seductive temptresses. But sadly, many young men and women drift toward each of these roles today.

Guys are so driven by their libidos (their sex drives) they will often do almost anything to fulfill them. Girls are often so desperate to find a guy who actually cares, they will sacrifice their own moral code to get one.

I like to ask my daughters, "What characteristics are you looking for in a husband?"

As they describe a perfect man, my guess is, they are *not* going to describe the kind of guy who only wants a girl if she gives him sex.

Girls, you are valuable! Don't lower your standards just because it seems like "the pickings are slim." Frankly, the pickings are often slim because you are looking in the wrong places.

Where do girls look for guys today? If they believe current popular songs, then they'll put on a tight dress, "drink it up," and "drop it low" at a nightclub. If they believe Scripture then they're going to devote themselves to fellowship among other things (Acts 2:42), and meet others who are devoted to Christ.

If you want to meet a godly man, hang out where godly men are. My daughters are both involved in ministry at their church, have gone on mission trips annually, and know numerous godly young men.

If a guy demands sex from you, he's not a guy worth having.

Is mutual masturbation okay?

Mutual masturbation is when couples stimulate themselves or each other without having intercourse. This is a sexual activity, and the Bible clearly says to avoid sexual activity like this until marriage. So don't do this unless you are married.

God's design for sex is always between a husband and wife. If a male or female ever masturbates while thinking about someone other than their spouse, that is lust, which is a sin. That's why married people should not watch porn together, because that causes them to lust for others, which is the same as inviting other people into their marriage bed.

Is a wet dream a sin?

When a young man has a nocturnal emission, is that a sin? Many teen boys are really embarrassed by these and don't want anyone to know. They wonder, *Did I sin in my sleep?*

No, I really don't think we can control our dreams. And wet dreams are a normal body function when guys get a buildup of semen. (Side note: Many guys never have wet dreams, because guys who masturbate regularly will probably rarely, if at all, have wet dreams.)

We can't control dreams, but we can, however, control what we fill our minds with. If we expose ourselves to sexual imagery, then our minds might dwell on some of that imagery. Control your thoughts during the day and your nights will most likely follow.

Wet dreams will still occur occasionally, and that's okay.

Why should I care if my looks or actions cause someone to lust? It's their own dirty mind, not my problem.

Believe it or not, some young people think like this. It's selfish and thoughtless. Consider these verses:

> Therefore let us stop passing judgment on one another. Instead, make up your mind not to put any stumbling block or obstacle in the way of a brother or sister.
>
> Romans 14:13 NIV

Let me ask you:

- What do the verses say we shouldn't do?
- What is a stumbling block?

- What are some of the ways those of the opposite sex stumble today?
- How can you avoid causing them to stumble?

Let us therefore make every effort to do what leads to peace and mutual edification.

Romans 14:19 NIV

Let me ask you:

- What are we to make every effort to do?
- What actions can we take that lead to peace and mutual edification?
- If someone has a dirty mind, what can we do to help edify them?

Is cohabitation okay?

This is a common question. I think this question gets answered when we truly seek to understand God's plan for sex and marriage. In other words, if we really study the Bible about God's plan for sex (chapter 1 of this book), how far we can go (chapter 2 of this book), and fleeing (chapter 3 of this book), then this question will answer itself. But many young people today haven't been educated with the truth; instead they've just been listening to the world's lies.

The world says, "You should test drive a car before you buy it. Couples should try living together to see if they are compatible."

The truth is, if a man and a woman each wait for sex until marriage, then seek to humbly serve each other (Ephesians 5), then sex and marriage are going to be amazing. Compatibility is for self-seeking individuals.

If two people move in together before marriage, the temptation will be to enjoy all the benefits of marriage without the commitment of marriage. This isn't God's plan and usually leads to pain and regret. In fact, couples who live together before marriage have a higher rate of divorce than couples who don't cohabitate before marriage.[3] Even more sobering, studies show that children of cohabiting couples are more likely to experience emotional problems, alcoholism, and drug abuse.[4] No one seems to know why, although experts speculate it might be because of the uncertainty of the relationship. In other words, the kids don't feel confident that Mom and Dad are really going to stick together. This has damaging effects.

Marriage vows often include the phrase "For better or worse." In other words, two people realize that there will be struggles when they are getting into a relationship. Conflict is a reality. Relationships take work, and hard work pays off. When two people enter a relationship with an attitude of "Let's try this, and we'll bail if it's difficult," the relationship is destined for failure. It's not a matter of *if* the relationship will fail . . . it's just a matter of *when*.

The "test drive" theory doesn't hold true. When Dad commits to Mom in marriage, it's better for their relationship and it's better for the kids.

How do I break out of an unhealthy cycle of sexual activity?

If you are asking this question, first, I applaud you for wanting to break this cycle. As we will discuss later in this chapter, Jesus doesn't care about your past, he cares about your future. So let's talk about how to break free of an unhealthy cycle of behavior.

If you want to break free of this unhealthy cycle of sexual activity, first determine if it's an addiction or just a habit of bad choices. If it's an addiction to porn, for example, you might want to see a counselor. This is nothing to be embarrassed of. An addiction is an addiction. (See chapter 4 for more about breaking free of porn.)

But if you have made a habit of sleeping with your girlfriend or boyfriend, then you can discover ways to flee this kind of temptation. You aren't alone, and in fact, most people endure this kind of temptation. But God is faithful to provide a way of escape (1 Corinthians 10:13).

Here's something to consider: Most choices began five choices ago.

Read that statement again and ponder it.

If you keep having sex with your boyfriend or girlfriend, my guess is it's not at school in algebra class. It's probably after school, at someone's house in a private place.

Ask yourself:

• Where are the places you are the most tempted?

• How can you avoid these places?

• Who is someone who can keep you accountable to doing this?

Maybe your unhealthy cycle of sexual activity is pornography and/or masturbation. If this is the case, read some of the tips we provided in chapter 4 on fleeing the grip of porn. This might mean asking Mom or Dad to add some porn filters in the house or get rid of some TV channels with distracting content. But this also should include talking with someone honestly about your struggles and asking for help.

The Bible constantly encourages us to enlist others in our journey.

Two people are better off than one, for they can help each other succeed. If one person falls, the other can reach out and help. But someone who falls alone is in real trouble.

Ecclesiastes 4:9–10

Don't go on this journey alone.

What if I don't get married? Does that mean I will never have sex, ever?!

The short answer: yes. Sex is for marriage. If you want to have sex, get married.

This isn't to say that remaining single is discouraged. In fact, the apostle Paul encouraged people to remain single if they were going to live a life of ministry. He says it like this:

I say this as a concession, not as a command. But I wish everyone were single, just as I am. Yet each person has a special gift from God, of one kind or another.

So I say to those who aren't married and to widows—it's better to stay unmarried, just as I am. But if they can't control themselves, they should go ahead and marry. It's better to marry than to burn with lust.

1 Corinthians 7:6–9

Paul was a missionary at heart. He traveled the world sharing the truth about Jesus, often getting arrested for standing up for truth. This was no life for a husband or father. That's why he wasn't afraid to give this personal little endorsement for staying single. He knew single people had more freedom to serve Jesus without any ties.

Yet, at the same time, Paul knew the power of lust. So he made it clear, "If they can't control themselves, they should go ahead and marry. It's better to marry than to burn with lust."

Singleness has its benefits. But if you want sex and intimacy, then enjoy it the way God intended it, in the relationship of marriage.

Is it wrong if I'm attracted to someone of the same sex?

This is just one of the many questions I've heard young people ask about homosexuality and same-sex attraction. Here are some other common questions:

What's wrong with homosexual activity? If God made people with a certain desire, why would he forbid them from it?

I don't like the opposite sex and I have feelings for the same sex. Does that mean I'm a homosexual?

If I had a homosexual experience but am still attracted to the opposite sex, does that make me bisexual?

I confess I was debating whether to even address this issue in this book. On one hand I know it's a common question that young people desperately need to hear truth about, but on the other hand, I know that the issue has grown so volatile that any answer on this issue divides people. So no matter what I write in these few pages, people are going to be looking for me to be one of two things: a *gay supporter*, or a *gay hater.*

If I had to choose one, I guess I'd have to be called a *gay supporter*, because I have gay friends and I love them. But I just happen to think that homosexual activity is a sin, just like looking at porn is a sin . . . as is lusting, cohabitating, and having premarital sex (not to mention gossiping, lying, and cheating on your taxes). Sadly, I have friends who are all of those things. Sadly, I am some of those things (in all honesty, I gossiped about someone last week). We all have something in common. We all need Jesus.

It's almost impossible to disagree with the homosexual lifestyle today without being labeled a hater. Questions about the issue are rarely asked without some emotion attached to them. Emotions are stirred because many who have experienced same-sex attraction have encountered teasing or bullying. Others might have kept these feelings to themselves but were afraid to ask questions. After all, the church has treated homosexuality as a uniquely terrible sin in the past. If you slept with your girlfriend or watched porn, that was one thing . . . but if you were gay? *Gasp!*

But the cultural climate has been changing rapidly in the last few years, and now homosexuality is almost completely accepted by the entertainment media community. If a celebrity were to speak out against homosexual behavior it would be career suicide. Movies, TV, and music frequently celebrate the homosexual lifestyle and are almost completely saturated with the message "How can something that feels so right be wrong?"

Rappers Macklemore and Ryan Lewis spoke the minds of many of today's young people with their song "Same Love" in 2012. This song not only spoke out against bullying (a good thing to protest); it also called out right-wing conservatives, saying they were paraphrasing a book written thousands of years ago, a clear "dis" on the Bible's clarity and relevance. The world readily accepts this message. In fact, the 2014 Grammys featured the rap duo performing this song while Queen Latifah officiated a mass gay wedding on the stage in front of millions of viewers.

Today, if anyone is asked what they think about the homosexual lifestyle, they dare not speak their minds if they don't agree with it. They don't want to be deemed intolerant or haters. As a result, many Christians are tiptoeing around the issue.

I don't tiptoe.

So I'll try to take the approach that Jesus took: *love* and *truth*. Jesus loved everyone, regardless of their sin; at the same time, he spoke the truth, even when it was very unpopular to do so.

Acting on Our Desires

Today the majority of young people think:

1. Homosexuals can't help but feel this way—they are "born this way."
2. We shouldn't judge them for feeling that way.
3. It's okay if they want to act on those desires.

Christians have been handling all three of these issues poorly. First, it's practically pointless to argue over number one, whether or not homosexuals are "born this way." This debate has never been settled either way, and frankly, it really doesn't need to be. Here's why: Desire isn't the issue—the issue is how we respond to our desires.

Think about it. We all know that some people are really prone to anger, some are prone to drinking, and some are really prone to lusting. Does that mean they should act out in these ways? Obviously not. I'm Irish and I have a really bad temper. Does that license me to go on tirades? Arguing about being "born this way" is really not relevant. The real issue is how I *act* on my desires.

Sadly, the church has been judging and mistreating homosexuals for years (number two above). This is ridiculous and against God's Word. First, we shouldn't judge any sinner; only God can judge. Most of the "correction" the Bible calls for is directed to believers in the church, and that is always supposed to be done in love. And as for condemning, even Jesus didn't come to condemn, but to save (John 3:17). It's silly that the church would be hung up pointing the finger at homosexuals when the church is full of gossips, porn addicts, and greedy people. The church needs to show love and grace like Jesus did.

But that doesn't mean we should swing the pendulum and say, "Okay then, homosexual activity is *not* a sin."

The fact is, the Bible makes it clear about God's design for sexual activity. It's something we've been talking about in this entire book, so it should come as no surprise: one man, one woman in the context of marriage. In fact, the Bible even goes as far as to speak out against homosexual activity specifically just as it speaks out against heterosexual sin. No, not just in the Old Testament, but in the New Testament as well.

For example, in 1 Corinthians 6:9–11 (NIV), we read:

> Do you not know that wrongdoers will not inherit the kingdom of God? Do not be deceived: Neither the sexually immoral nor idolaters nor adulterers nor men who have sex with men nor thieves nor the greedy nor drunkards nor slanderers nor swindlers will inherit the kingdom of God. And that is what some of you were. But you were washed, you were sanctified, you were justified in the name of the Lord Jesus Christ and by the Spirit of our God.

In this passage, Paul is unmistakably condemning certain sins, with homosexuality being one of them—right along with greed and drunkenness—lest we think that one sinful lifestyle is worse (or better) than another. These are things Christians shouldn't be doing.

While some may want to see this passage as just another "clobber verse," it is best viewed as a passage of supreme hope! Look for yourselves. Notice that the passage says, "And that is what some of you were."

Were.

Instead of remaining in their sin, the Corinthians were washed, sanctified, and justified in the name of Jesus and by the power of God's Spirit! That's because God loves idolaters, adulterers, drunkards, thieves, slanderers, swindlers, and yes, homosexuals! I'm glad God's process of sanctification is at work in my life, because I'm really good at slandering people who make me mad. It's an area I've really needed to give to God, and he's slowly changing me.

In another of Paul's references to homosexuality, in 1 Timothy 1:9–11, he says,

> The law was not intended for people who do what is right. It is for people who are lawless and rebellious, who are ungodly and sinful, who consider nothing sacred and defile what is holy, who kill their father or mother or commit other murders. The law is for people who are sexually immoral, or who practice homosexuality, or are slave traders, liars, promise breakers, or who do anything else that contradicts the wholesome teaching that comes from the glorious Good News entrusted to me by our blessed God.

Here Paul lists those "who practice homosexuality" among the "lawless and rebellious." It is point blank doctrine: Homosexuality is a lifestyle that's contradictory to the Gospel. But look what else Paul is doing. He's also clearly saying that God has reached out to the "lawless and rebellious" with his perfect law. Rather than condemn them, *God desires to redeem them*!

Romans chapter 1 paints it pretty plainly as well as Paul describes some of the shameful things mankind does, trading the truth about God for a lie:

> That is why God abandoned them to their shameful desires. Even the women turned against the natural way to have sex and instead indulged in sex with each other. And the men, instead of having normal sexual relations with women, burned with lust for each other. Men did shameful things with other men,

and as a result of this sin, they suffered within themselves the penalty they deserved.

vv. 26–27

The whole chapter is pretty clear that homosexual activity was not God's intent. It also details some other sins like greed, envy, and quarreling. (Funny, no one seems to be arguing that those actions are okay.)

While the Bible's mention of homosexuality seems completely straightforward, many argue that when the Bible uses the word *homosexual* it really means something else. Some argue that when the apostle Paul discusses homosexuality in 1 Corinthians 6:9 or 1 Timothy 1:10, what he was *really* denouncing was pederasty, the sexual abuse of boys by men, which was sometimes practiced by Roman and Greek citizens.

I have just one question: *Then why didn't Paul just say that?* You see, the apostle Paul was a man of profound specifics, who at times would even invent words to get his point across, like the concept of "justification" (Romans 4 and 5). Am I to believe that he simply began to use terms that were generic or vague or *even wrong* when talking about such important issues?

If Paul wanted to address adult-to-child sin, he would have done that. He didn't. The reason he didn't speak of pederasty was because he was referring to homosexuality.

But don't forget that these passages are all in the context of God's grace. All the passages above clearly communicate God's love for us and our need for his forgiveness. All of us need this love and grace.

If we're struggling with desires to engage in homosexual activity, we need to resist that temptation, just like those who are struggling with lust, porn, or any heterosexual sin. (Read more about fleeing sexual sin in the previous chapters.) Yes, most of us are in the same boat, struggling with these temptations, and we need Jesus badly.

How Do We Answer Our Friends if They Ask Us About This Issue?

1. UNDERSTAND WHERE YOUR FRIENDS ARE COMING FROM.

Remember to ask a lot of questions. If your friend asks, "Is it wrong to be gay?" Ask them, "That's a good question. Tell me more about why you're asking." Gather as much information as possible so you can be sensitive to their feelings. Ask them, "What do you think?" Remember this is a very emotional issue for many.

2. SHARE GOD'S AMAZING PLAN FOR SEX AND MARRIAGE.

Don't jump straight to a passage listing homosexuals among the immoral. Tell them God's story of how he created a husband and wife and told them to enjoy sex together (much of what you read in chapter 1). Help them understand God's plan and what happens when people go outside of God's plan. Remember that many young people don't see the Bible as an authority. So be prepared to discuss it beyond just "because the Bible says so."

3. SHARE JESUS' LOVE FOR "SINNERS LIKE ME."

One of the biggest reasons the world dislikes Christians is because some Christians come across as hateful and judgmental. Christ was neither of these things. In fact, Jesus claimed countless times that he came to save sinners. Help your friend understand that you need Jesus just like every sinner needs Jesus.

4. HELP THEM UNDERSTAND THAT ALL SEXUAL SIN IS OUTSIDE OF GOD'S PLAN.

If your friend wants to specifically know if you think homosexual activity is a sin, talk about homosexuality in the context of other sexual sins. Start by asking about other sexual sins. If a teenage boy really wants to sleep with his girlfriend, is it okay? Why not? If it feels right, how could it be wrong? If a man really wants to look at porn, can he? Why not? But he loves looking at naked women, how could that be wrong? What if they are underage women? Couldn't it be argued that he was born with these desires?

So should we follow every desire we have? What about desires for the same sex? The world loves to tell us that we should follow our every desire, but the truth is, sometimes our desires are sinful. We need to learn to follow God, not every desire (Galatians 5:16–17).

Our world is confused by this messy issue. Sadly, homosexuals have been bullied. This is a tragedy. It should have never happened. Sadly, homosexuals have been judged and singled out. This has made it very difficult for those struggling with same-sex attraction.

As Christians, we need to love the homosexual just like we need to love a porn addict or the unmarried heterosexual couple cohabitating next door. When we model this kind of love, others will be attracted to Christ's love in us.

Pray through this whole process. Pray specifically that God will help you live out these principles and answer these questions in love and truth. And remember, our love will point to truth loudly.

I've already had sex; why bother to save myself anymore?

This is such a common question among young people. Sadly, many of us have a blotted past and think, *I'm already damaged goods.*

Past imperfections don't impede fresh futures . . . especially when Jesus offers us a new beginning!

If you read the Gospels, you'll notice that imperfect people seemed especially attracted to Jesus. In fact, the more messed up they were, the more they wanted to meet this guy Jesus, who offered repentance and a fresh start. In story after story you'll see it. A scam artist named Zacchaeus (Luke 19), a promiscuous woman Jesus met at a well (John 4), even a criminal on the cross next to him (Luke 23). They all had made really huge mistakes in their past, and Jesus forgave them, only concerned about their future.

One of the best examples of this was in John chapter 8 when the Pharisees brought Jesus a woman caught in the act of adultery, demanding he tell them what to do with her. Instead of accusing her, he put the attention on the accusers, saying, "All right, but let the one who has never sinned throw the first stone!" (John 8:7).

The accusers all left one at a time, and Jesus finally asked her,

"Didn't even one of them condemn you?"

"No, Lord," she said.

And Jesus said, "Neither do I. Go and sin no more."

John 8:10–11

Jesus doesn't care about your past, but he cares about your future. First John 1:8–9 spells it out:

If we claim we have no sin, we are only fooling ourselves and not living in the truth. But if we confess our sins to him, he is faithful and just to forgive us our sins and to cleanse us from all wickedness.

Jesus offers us a fresh start. He is willing to cleanse us from our past mistakes.

But don't let past missteps justify future mistakes. God's grace isn't a license to continue to sin.

Sometimes when we hear about how compassionate and forgiving God is, we use that as an excuse to sin even more. *After all, I can just ask for forgiveness later.*

This can hurt us two ways.

First, and foremost, it hurts our relationship with God. The foundation of our relationship with God is based on our trust in him. How much are we trusting in him if we aren't willing to give everything to him?

Paul tackles this faulty logic in Romans chapter 6. He asks,

> Well then, should we keep on sinning so that God can show us more and more of his wonderful grace? Of course not! Since we have died to sin, how can we continue to live in it?
>
> Romans 6:1–2

Paul goes on to urge us to put our complete trust in God, warning, "Do not let sin control the way you live; do not give in to sinful desires" (v. 12).

Second, using past missteps as an excuse to justify future mistakes can also bring some pretty severe consequences upon ourselves. God is willing to forgive us, but that doesn't necessarily free us from natural consequences.

If a teenager gets his girlfriend pregnant, God's forgiveness doesn't free him from the ramifications of that decision.

If a teenage girl gets chlamydia and never realizes she has it (which happens frequently because the disease is asymptomatic), the consequences are often infertility.

Our choices have consequences. God's grace isn't a "get out of jail free" card for natural consequences.

Don't let past imperfections prevent fresh futures . . . especially when Jesus offers us a new beginning.

So what do you do if you are tempted again? What do you do if you feel guilt or shame from a past mistake?

1. Ask God for his help. Pray and specifically ask him for forgiveness and help to make positive choices today and tomorrow.

2. Talk with someone you trust. Talk with a parent, mentor, or trusted friend about your mistake. The Bible encourages us to "confess your sins to each other" so we can be healed (James 5:16). When we share our dark past with caring people, they can encourage us and hold us accountable to a bright future.

What if I've been abused or raped?

First, understand you are not alone.

According to recent studies by David Finkelhor, Director of the Crimes Against Children Research Center:

- One in five girls and one in twenty boys is a victim of child sexual abuse.

- Twenty-eight percent of U.S. youth ages fourteen to seventeen said they had been sexually victimized at some time in their lives.

- Children are most vulnerable to sexual abuse between the ages of seven and thirteen.[5]

According to a 2003 National Institute of Justice report, three out of four adolescents who have been sexually assaulted were victimized by someone they knew well.[6]

Young people carrying the burden of sexual abuse often feel dirty or used. Sadly, they might even feel it is their own fault. If you have been sexually assaulted or victimized, let me assure you, you're not alone and it's not your fault. So let me recommend three steps that can help you navigate this painful past:

Report It

Sometimes people avoid reporting abuse because of the pain and embarrassment, but this often leaves a predator free to do more harm. Most sexual predators act repeatedly. Your reporting could prevent countless future victims from the abuse or victimization you endured. I know it's very difficult to talk to someone about something so painful or embarrassing, but telling someone is often the first step on a road to healing. If you don't know how or where, tell a teacher or a principal, or . . . step two can help you with that.

Seek Professional Help

This isn't something you should be embarrassed about. Counselors can provide the tools individuals need to overcome past hurt. They can also provide some guidance to help you heal.

Focus on the Future

Don't dwell on a painful past when Jesus offers us such a bright future. As a victim, we often blame ourselves and focus on the past. God doesn't care about your past; he cares about your future.

This kind of hurt is never easy. There is no magic Band-Aid that makes it all better after one application. Healing takes time. So when you feel hopeless or ashamed, remember the two tips I shared in my answer to the last question:

1. Ask God for his help. Pray and specifically ask him for deliverance from feelings of guilt and shame.

2. Talk with someone you trust. Talk with a parent, mentor, or trusted friend about your past. Let them know your feelings. Sometimes you can even find recovery groups full of people with similar life experiences.

God can carry you through these tough times. Some of us don't reach out to him until we need him, but that doesn't stop him from being there.

Corrie ten Boom, a wise woman imprisoned for helping Jews escape the Nazi Holocaust, said, "You may never know that Jesus is all you need, until Jesus is all you have."

Jesus offers a fresh start for everyone.

Everyone.

Discussion Questions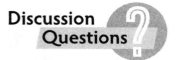

1. Which one of the questions in this chapter is a question you would have asked? Did you like the answer? Explain.
2. Which one of these questions is the most common question you think your friends would have today? Why?
3. How would you answer if they asked you that question?
4. In this chapter we discussed past mistakes. Why do you think people have trouble letting go of past mistakes?
5. Read the following passage of Scripture:

Therefore, since we are surrounded by such a huge crowd of witnesses to the life of faith, let us strip off every weight that slows us down, especially the sin that so easily trips us up. And let us run with endurance the race God has set before us. We do this by keeping our eyes on Jesus, the champion who initiates and perfects our faith. Because of the joy awaiting him, he endured the cross, disregarding its shame. Now he is seated in the place of honor beside God's throne.

Hebrews 12:1–2

What does the first verse tell us to "strip off"?

6. What might be slowing you down or tripping you up in your life journey?

7. What does the verse tell us to focus on as we run with endurance?

8. How can you keep your eyes on Jesus today, this week, this month?

9. What is something you can do this week to make this possible?

10. What can a caring friend or adult mentor do to help you with this?

Finale

The Journey

What now?

That's the question many of us have to ask at this point.

Think about it. So far, we've examined three truths in depth:

1. God's design really does make sense. No matter which way we look at it, it seems that sex is the most enjoyable in a marriage relationship where two people are loving each other and selflessly seeking to meet each other's needs.

2. Moments of intimacy are clearly designed for marriage. These moments are difficult to stop . . . *because they're not supposed to be stopped*. In fact, we shouldn't start these moments until marriage, when we can enjoy them with the one person we'll share them with uniquely for a lifetime.

3. Pornography and sexually charged entertainment media provoke lust, and lusting is just like committing adultery against our future spouse. We need to flee any temptations that cause us to lust or engage in sexual immorality.

These facts seem clear. The question is, *What are we going to do with this information?*

Recalculating

Some of us might be wondering, *What if it's too late?* In other words, *What if I've already messed up?*

I briefly answered that question in the previous chapter, but it's worth addressing again. Jesus offers a fresh start for everyone.

Everyone.

Have you ever veered off the path while on a road trip? Ever taken a wrong turn?

There is one word a GPS uses that we all know too well: *recalculating.*

I might be driving to Los Angeles, but when I turn off the freeway to grab a Wendy's Frosty, a soft female voice calmly says, "Recalculating."

If road construction sends you miles off course and you have no idea where you are, the word *recalculating* actually brings hope. It's a voice that says, "I haven't given up. Sure, we've veered from our intended course, but I'm still going to get you there. Let's start again from this new location."

It would be pretty discouraging if our GPS said, "Pull over and shut off the ignition; you have passed the point of no return. This is where you are going to die."

My GPS has never done that. Instead . . . "Recalculating."

In other words, "Don't give up. We'll get there."

Maybe you've made some mistakes in your past. You're not alone. Me too. I'm still paying for some of them, but I'm not letting those mistakes define me. Jesus doesn't care about our past, he cares about our future. Past imperfections don't impede fresh futures.

So what are your plans for your future in the area of sex and intimacy?

Maybe you've already learned some lessons. That's okay. How can you take that knowledge and use it for a better future?

Your choices today determine your tomorrow.

Worth the Wait

As you look at your options, you could take the easy route that so many are taking . . . or you could put your faith in God and follow his design. One route focuses on the immediate thrill, but has long-term consequences. The other way takes discipline for a few years, followed by a lifetime of the most enjoyable sex.

When I was young it seemed like I was going to have to wait forever to get married. That handful of years seemed to move by so slowly. But after you have been married for twenty years, the few years before you were married truly seem like nothing. In fact:

- You have a whole lifetime to have lots of great sex, and saving yourself for marriage will only make that lifetime of sex better.

- If you and your spouse are seeking to meet each other's needs as God intended, then you will also be having more sex than your "promiscuous" friends . . . a lot more sex.

- You will also be having better sex, the most enjoyable sex, actually. Sex without guilt, regret, or fear.

The answer is simply *discipline*. Your discipline now is a gift to your future spouse. All you are doing is trading a few years of *discipline* for a lifetime of *awesome* connecting in ways you probably can't even imagine yet.

What is your first step in this journey?

Do you have someone you can talk with about this, a parent or trusted mentor? Begin the conversation. In a world full of explicit lies, it's good to have someone who is not afraid to talk with you explicitly about the truth.

Notes

Chapter 1: Why Wait?

1. "Nationally Representative CDC Study Finds 1 in 4 Teenage Girls Has a Sexually Transmitted Disease," Centers for Disease Control and Prevention, March 10, 2008, www.cdc.gov/stdconference/2008/press/release-11march2008.htm.

2. "HPV and Cancer," National Cancer Institute at the National Institutes of Health, www.cancer.gov/cancertopics/factsheet/Risk/HPV.

3. Dr. Ricki Pollycove, "Condoms Not Effective Against HPV or Herpes," SFGate, http://m.sfgate.com/health/article/Condoms-not-effective-against-HPV-or-herpes-3650285.php.

4. "Chlamydia—CDC Fact Sheet," Centers for Disease Control and Prevention, January 2013, www.cdc.gov/Std/chlamydia/STDFact-Chlamydia.htm.

5. Ross Douthat, "Why Monogamy Matters," *The New York Times*, March 6, 2011, www.nytimes.com/2011/03/07/opinion/07douthat.html?_r=0.

6. E.O. Laumann, J.H. Gagnon, R.T. Michael, and S. Michaels, *The Social Organization of Sexuality: Sexual Practices in the United States* (Chicago: The University of Chicago Press, 1994).

7. Ibid., 115.

8. Ibid.

9. R. J. Levin and A. Levin, "Sexual Pleasure: The Surprising Preferences of 100,000 Women," *Redbook*, September 1975, 51–58.

10. David G. Blanchflower and Andrew J. Oswald, *Money, Sex, and Happiness: An Empirical Study* (National Bureau of Economic Research Working Paper No. 10499, May 2004), cited in David R. Francis, "Monogamy Is Good—And Good For You," *The Christian Science Monitor,* December 5, 2005, www.csmonitor.com/2005/1205/p15s01-cogn.html.

11. Mark D. White, Ph.D., "On Monogamy, Happiness, and Adultery," *Psychology Today*, March 12, 2011, www.psychologytoday.com/blog/maybe-its-just-me/201103/monogamy-happiness-and-adultery.

12. Maia Szalavitz, "How Oxytocin Makes Men (Almost) Monogamous," *Time*, November 27, 2013, http://healthland.time.com/2013/11/27/how-oxytocin-makes-men-almost-monogamous.

13. "HPV and Cancer," National Cancer Institute at the National Institutes of Health, www.cancer.gov/cancertopics/factsheet/Risk/HPV.

14. "Abortion Facts," National Abortion Federation, www.prochoice.org/education-and-advocacy-about_abortion/abortion-facts.

Chapter 3: Fleeing

1. "Dirty Song Lyrics Can Prompt Early Teen Sex," NBCnews.com, August 7, 2006, www.nbcnews.com/id/14227775/ns/health-sexual_health/t/dirty-song-lyrics-can-prompt-early-teen-sex.

2. Rebecca Hagelin, "Study Shows Teens Imitate Risky Sex of Films, TV," *The Washington Times,* August 12, 2012, www.washingtontimes.com/news/2012/aug/12/hagelin-study-shows-teens-imitate-risky-sex-of-fil/#ixzz2gUzHLlc0.

3. "Report of the APA Task Force on the Sexualization of Girls: Executive Summary," American Psychological Association, 2007, www.apa.org/pi/wpo/sexualization.html.

4. "Freshman Women's Binge Drinking Tied to Sexual Assault Risk," *Science Blog*, December 8, 2011, http://scienceblog.com/50305/freshman-womens-binge-drinking-tied-to-sexual-assault-risk, citing Testa, M., & Hoffman, J. H. (January 2012). "Naturally Occurring Changes in Women's Drinking From High School to College and Implications for Sexual Victimization," *Journal of Studies on Alcohol and Drugs,* 73(1), 26.

Chapter 4: The Lure of Porn and Masturbation

1. "Children and Pornography," Center for Parent/Youth Understanding, www.digitalkidsinitiative.com/files/2014/08/Children_and_Pornography_Factsheet-Revised-August-2014.pdf

2. "Pornography Statistics" Covenant Eyes, www.covenanteyes.com/pornstats.

3. Ibid.

4. "Internet Porn Making Men Bad in Bed," *International Business Times*, October 24, 2011, www.ibtimes.co.uk/Internet-porn-making-men-bad-in-bed-porn-xxx-pornography-sex-sexual-intercourse-cam2cam-erectile-dys-236295.

5. M. Robinson and G. Wilson, "Cupid's Poisoned Arrow: Porn-Induced Sexual Dysfunction Growing Problem," *Psychology Today,* July 11, 2011.

6. Ibid.

7. Alan Mozes, "Study Tracks Masturbation Trends Among U.S. Teens," *U.S. News and World Report*, August 1, 2011, http://health.usnews.com/health-news/family-health/womens-health/articles/2011/08/01/study-tracks-masturbation-trends-among-us-teens.

8. "Millennials in Adulthood," PewResearch, March 7, 2014, www.pewsocial trends.org/2014/03/07/millennials-in-adulthood.

9. Jordan Monge, "The Real Problem With Female Masturbation," *Christianity Today*, April 2014, www.christianitytoday.com/women/2014/april/real-problem -with-female-masturbation.html.

10. John Piper, "ANTHEM: Strategies for Fighting Lust," Desiring God, November 5, 2001, www.desiringgod.org/articles/anthem-strategies-for-fighting-lust.

Chapter 5: Tough Questions

1. Randye Hoder, "Study Finds Most Teens Sext Before They're 18," *Time*, July 3, 2014, http://time.com/2948467/chances-are-your-teen-is-sexting.

2. Dr. Sanjay Gupta, "Have You Had the 'Sext' Talk with Your Kids?" CNN Health, June 30, 2014, http://thechart.blogs.cnn.com/2014/06/30/have-you-had-the-sext-talk-with-your-kids.

3. Casey E. Copen, Ph.D.; Kimberly Daniels, Ph.D.; Jonathan Vespa, Ph.D.; and William D. Mosher, Ph.D., *First Marriages in the United States: Data From the 2006–2010 National Survey of Family Growth*, National Health Statistics Reports, No. 49, March 22, 2012, 2, www.cdc.gov/nchs/data/nhsr/nhsr049.pdf.

4. Sharon Jayson, "Living Together: No Big Deal?" *USA Today*, March 26, 2011, http://usatoday30.usatoday.com/printedition/life/20080609/d_worldcohab09 .art.htm.

5. "Child Sexual Abuse Statistics," The National Center for Victims of Crime, www.victimsofcrime.org/media/reporting-on-child-sexual-abuse/child -sexual-abuse-statistics.

6. Dean G. Kilpatrick, Benjamin E. Saunders, and Daniel W. Smith, *Youth Victimization: Prevalence and Implications* (Washington, D.C.: U.S. Department of Justice, 2003), 5.

Jonathan McKee is an expert on youth culture and the author of more than a dozen books, including *The Zombie Apocalypse Survival Guide for Teenagers* and *The Guy's Guide to God, Girls, and the Phone in Your Pocket*. He has twenty years of youth-ministry experience and speaks to parents and leaders worldwide. He also writes about parenting and youth culture while providing free resources at TheSource4Parents.com. Jonathan, his wife, Lori, and their three kids live in California.

JonathanMcKeeWrites.com
Twitter.com/InJonathansHead